T0323242

Critical Thinking and Reflection for Mental Health Nursing Students

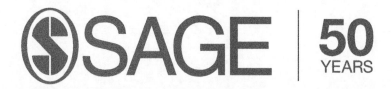

SAGE was founded in 1965 by Sara Miller McCune to support the dissemination of usable knowledge by publishing innovative and high-quality research and teaching content. Today, we publish more than 850 journals, including those of more than 300 learned societies, more than 800 new books per year, and a growing range of library products including archives, data, case studies, reports, and video. SAGE remains majority-owned by our founder, and after Sara's lifetime will become owned by a charitable trust that secures our continued independence.

Los Angeles | London | New Delhi | Singapore | Washington DC

Critical Thinking and Reflection for Mental Health Nursing Students

Marc Roberts

s Angeles | London | New Delhi
gapore | Washington DC

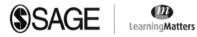

Learning Matters
An imprint of SAGE Publications Ltd
1 Oliver's Yard
55 City Road
London EC1Y 1SP

SAGE Publications Inc.
2455 Teller Road
Thousand Oaks, California 91320

SAGE Publications India Pvt Ltd
B 1/I 1 Mohan Cooperative Industrial Area
Mathura Road
New Delhi 110 044

SAGE Publications Asia-Pacific Pte Ltd
3 Church Street
#10-04 Samsung Hub
Singapore 049483

First published 2015

Library of Congress Control Number: 2015948016

British Library Cataloguing in Publication Data

A catalogue record for this book is available from the British Library

Editor: Alex Clabburn
Development editor: Eleanor Rivers
Production controller: Chris Marke
Project management: Swales & Willis Ltd, Exeter, Devon
Marketing manager: Tamara Navaratnam
Cover design: Wendy Scott
Typeset by: C&M Digitals (P) Ltd, Chennai, India
Printed and bound by CPI Group (UK) Ltd, Croydon, CR0 4YY

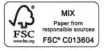

ISBN 978-1-4739-1311-0
ISBN 978-1-4739-1312-7 (pbk)

Contents

Transforming Nursing Practice is a series tailor-made for pre-registration student nurses. Each book in the series is:

○ Affordable
○ Mapped to the NMC Standards and Essential Skills Clusters
○ Full of active learning features
○ Focused on applying theory to practice

Each book addresses a core topic and they have been carefully developed to be simple to use, quick to read and written in clear language.

> " An invaluable series of books that explicitly relates to the NMC standards. Each book cover a different topic that students need to explore in order to develop into a qualified nurse... I would recommend this series to all Pre-Registration nursing students whatever their field or year of study
>
> **Linda Robson**
> **Senior Lecturer, Edge Hill University**
>
> The set of books is an excellent resource for students. The series is small, easily portable and valuable. I use the whole set on a regular basis.
>
> **Fiona Davies**
> **Senior Nurse Lecturer, University of Derby**
>
> I recommend the SAGE/Learning Matters series to all my students as they are relevant and concise. Please keep up the good work.
>
> **Thomas Beary**
> **Senior Lecturer in Mental Health Nursing, University of Hertfordshire** "

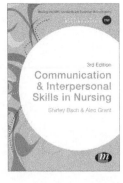

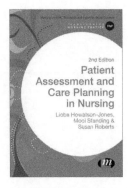

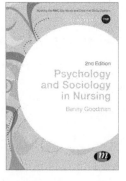

ABOUT THE SERIES EDITORS

Professor Shirley Bach is now retired and was formerly Head of the School of Health Sciences at the University of Brighton and responsible for the core knowledge titles. Previously she was head of post-graduate studies and has developed curriculum for undergraduate and pre-registration courses in a variety of subject domains.

Dr Mooi Standing is an independent academic consultant (UK and International) and responsible for the personal and professional learning skills titles. She is an accredited NMC quality assurance reviewer of educational programmes and a professional regulator panellist on the NMC Practice Committee.

Sandra Walker is Senior Teaching Fellow in Mental Health at the University of Southampton and responsible for the mental health nursing titles. She is a qualified mental health nurse with a wide range of clinical experience spanning more than 20 years.

CORE KNOWLEDGE TITLES:

Becoming a Registered Nurse: Making the Transition to Practice
Communication and Interpersonal Skills in Nursing (3rd Ed)
Contexts of Contemporary Nursing (2nd Ed)
Getting into Nursing (2nd Ed)
Health Promotion and Public Health for Nursing Students (2nd Ed)
Introduction to Medicines Management in Nursing
Law and Professional Issues in Nursing (3rd Ed)
Leadership, Management and Team Working in Nursing (2nd Ed)
Learning Skills for Nursing Students
Medicines Management in Children's Nursing
Nursing and Collaborative Practice (2nd Ed)
Nursing and Mental Health Care
Nursing in Partnership with Patients and Carers
Passing Calculations Tests for Nursing Students (3rd Ed)
Palliative and End of Life Care in Nursing
Patient Assessment and Care Planning in Nursing (2nd Ed)
Patient and Carer Participation in Nursing
Patient Safety and Managing Risk in Nursing
Psychology and Sociology in Nursing (2nd Ed)
Successful Practice Learning for Nursing Students (2nd Ed)
Understanding Ethics in Nursing Practice
Using Health Policy in Nursing
What is Nursing? Exploring Theory and Practice (3rd Ed)

PERSONAL AND PROFESSIONAL LEARNING SKILLS TITLES:

Clinical Judgement and Decision Making for Nursing Students (2nd Ed)
Critical Thinking and Writing for Nursing Students (3rd Ed)
Evidence-based Practice in Nursing (2nd Ed)
Information Skills for Nursing Students
Reflective Practice in Nursing (3rd Ed)
Succeeding in Essays, Exams & OSCEs for Nursing Students
Succeeding in Literature Reviews and Research Project Plans for Nursing Students (2nd Ed)
Successful Professional Portfolios for Nursing Students (2nd Ed)
Understanding Research for Nursing Students (2nd Ed)

MENTAL HEALTH NURSING TITLES:

Assessment and Decision Making in Mental Health Nursing
Engagement and Therapeutic Communication in Mental Health Nursing
Medicines Management in Mental Health Nursing
Mental Health Law in Nursing
Physical Healthcare and Promotion in Mental Health Nursing
Psychosocial Interventions in Mental Health Nursing

ADULT NURSING TITLES:

Acute and Critical Care in Adult Nursing
Caring for Older People in Nursing
Medicines Management in Adult Nursing
Nursing Adults with Long Term Conditions (2nd Ed)
Safeguarding Adults in Nursing Practice
Dementia Care in Nursing

You can find more information on each of these titles and our other learning resources at **www.sagepub.co.uk**. Many of these titles are also available in various e-book formats, please visit our website for more information.

Foreword

When I started out as a mental health nursing student in the 1980s I had a naive expectation that everything that went on in the care of mental health patients was the best quality, the most effective and the best for the patient. It did not take me long to realise that, in this ever-increasingly complex world of mental health, this was not the case. It was only over time though, as I developed my ability to think critically and not accept at face value the information that comes from all sources around you as a nurse, that I became a more competent practitioner. It is not that long ago, historically speaking, that we were advocating deep insulin comas, ice-cold baths and other, now considered barbaric, practices in an effort to help people manage their mental health. If people had not questioned these practices perhaps they would still be in use today. Critical thinking is one of the most essential development tools you can foster; it is extremely important for the safety of patients in making sure that the care they receive is the least restrictive and truly effective for them.

A particular area of concern in mental health care is the social control element of the service. This is long-standing and it is here, often, that we still see questionable practice 'done to' people despite clear indications from them that this is not what they need. The very existence of the Mental Health Act is often challenged and at odds with some of the Human Rights Act. In these complex times the art of thinking critically is ever more important and *Critical Thinking and Reflection for Mental Health Nursing Students* provides a comprehensive introduction to the subject.

This book not only introduces you to the concept of critical thinking, reflection and practice – it also encourages you to think more widely about the idea of 'other'. Through the sensitively created exercises throughout the book you are encouraged to think more deeply about many contentious issues, including the role of the media in perpetuating prejudice, and how stigma is often inherent in our practice in the 'us and them' attitude we can find ourselves taking without thinking. The author encourages us to consider ways in which we can address this stigma when we notice it in both ourselves, via closer observation of self-awareness practices, and others, by challenging it in gentle but effective ways.

If you are a student nurse, a newly qualified nurse or even a nurse of some years' standing looking for tips to update your portfolio of skills, *Critical Thinking and Reflection for Mental Health Nursing Students* will stand you in good stead for practice. It can be read as a whole, but can also be dipped into section by section as you come across situations in your journey that warrant further exploration or practice of that particular subject. Engaging with this book will help you to become a more effective practitioner of the art of mental health nursing, enhancing your ability to provide effective care for people of diverse backgrounds and needs as well as enhancing your ability to write academically.

In the opening sentence of this book, the author states that there has never been a more exciting time to become a mental health nurse. I believe he is right.

Sandra Walker

Series Editor

About the author

Dr Marc Roberts is an independent researcher and writer with extensive and varied experience working in mental health practice and education. In addition to being a registered mental health nurse, he is also a professional philosopher whose research is concerned with the manner in which critical thinking, critical reflection and philosophy more generally can contribute to the theory and practice of contemporary mental health care.

Acknowledgements

I would like to thank Becky Taylor for her work in commissioning this book, Eleanor Rivers for her valuable contributions throughout its development and Sandra Walker for her supportive reading of the original drafts. In addition, I wish to thank Robin Ion and the staff and students at the Centre of Excellence in Mental Health Nursing and Counselling at Abertay University, Dundee for the stimulating critical questions and discussions about all aspects of contemporary mental health care that inspired the present work. Finally, I would like to thank Philippa, Ruth and John for their encouragement, support and patience throughout the writing process.

Introduction

Who is this book for?

This book is written primarily for mental health nursing students currently undertaking their pre-registration training. However, it may also be of interest to qualified mental health nurses who wish to develop or refresh their critical thinking and reflection skills. In addition, those involved in the education of mental health nursing students, such as lecturers and clinical mentors, might find the book a useful resource for relevant teaching, learning and assessment activities.

Why *Critical Thinking and Reflection for Mental Health Nursing Students*?

Contemporary mental health care is an exciting, challenging and changing field. Established practices and traditional ways of understanding mental health and distress are being challenged, both by those who work within and those who use contemporary mental health services. The authority of mental health professionals and the legitimacy of their interventions are open to question as never before, and those who use mental health services are increasingly calling for greater involvement in how their experiences are understood and addressed. In this changing and challenging environment, the roles that you will be required to perform as a qualified mental health nurse are becoming increasingly sophisticated. Not only will you be expected to identify, evaluate and apply various forms of information, research and evidence to your mental health practice, but you will be expected to work in a recovery-focused way with those who use mental health services and this will require an awareness of how your own assumptions, values and beliefs may affect your practice in both productive and non-productive ways. Contemporary mental health nursing therefore demands that you become an informed, self-aware and proactive mental health professional and central to achieving this is the ability to engage in critical thinking and critical reflection. This book will enable you to begin to develop your critical thinking and reflective capabilities for your work in both the clinical and university setting and, importantly, it will do so by situating critical thinking and reflection in the context of the debates, challenges and changes that characterise contemporary mental health care.

Book structure

Chapter 1 introduces you to critical thinking in mental health nursing. While critical thinking is to be understood as a complex and multidimensional activity, a provisional definition of critical thinking is provided and the significance and importance of thinking critically in contemporary mental health nursing is considered. In order to develop and deepen that understanding of critical thinking, the chapter also examines the manner in which critical thinking requires not only the employment of certain intellectual skills but also the possession of a number of emotional attributes or personal qualities.

Chapter 2 is concerned with critical reflection in mental health nursing. In particular, a provisional definition of critical reflection is provided, before highlighting the benefits of that activity and discussing its significance for you as a mental health nursing student and throughout your subsequent career as a mental health nurse. While a variety of models and frameworks have been devised in order to assist the process of reflection, the chapter examines three underlying principles and stages that will help you to understand and engage in the activity of critical reflection.

Chapter 3 considers the notion of critical mental health practice and enables you to begin to think about how you can develop such practice. In doing so, it focuses upon the manner in which your engagement in critical thinking and reflection may be limited by a variety of personal, social and institutional obstacles. While you may encounter multiple and diverse challenges to such critical activity, the chapter examines four in particular that can be understood as being representative of the variety of obstacles that can potentially limit the incorporation of critical thinking and critical reflection into your mental health practice.

Chapter 4 is concerned with the notion of values and values-based practice in mental health nursing. As well as encouraging you to consider critically your personal values and the professional values of mental health nursing, it examines the importance of working with the values of those who use mental health services. In addition, the chapter introduces you to one of the most enduring and significant critical discussions surrounding the role of values in contemporary mental health care and, in particular, the role that values play in understanding, conceptualising and responding to mental distress.

Chapter 5 discusses the manner in which those who experience mental distress have often been thought of as being different from the rest of society's members and, as a consequence of that difference, have been subject to stigma, prejudice and discrimination. However, as well as discussing the general processes by which people who experience mental distress can be subject to practices of exclusion – and designated as different or 'other' – the chapter also examines the manner in which stigma, prejudice and discrimination can be understood as affecting different groups of mental health service users in different ways.

Chapter 6 introduces you to various critical debates surrounding the interventions that are used in contemporary mental health care and the involvement of those people who use mental health services in that care. In particular, the chapter examines a number of critical discussions that are concerned with the use of physical and psychological interventions in contemporary mental health care, as well as critical questions about service user involvement and the extent to which a recovery-orientated approach can be reconciled with the range of responsibilities that mental health services are expected to meet.

Chapter 7 considers the standards against which academic work generally, and your critical thinking and reflective capabilities in particular, can be assessed. While a variety of academic standards exist, the chapter examines three standards that are commonly employed to assess the content of academic work and three standards that are commonly employed to assess the form of academic work. Throughout the chapter you are encouraged to think about, and work in accordance with, these standards in order to begin to develop your ability to produce high-quality academic assignments for your mental health nursing programme.

Chapter 8 examines a series of questions that can be used to evaluate critically the large amount of information that you will encounter during your mental health nursing programme. In particular, it discusses the importance of asking six critically evaluative questions of any piece of information to which you will be introduced, or that you may access, in both the university and clinical setting. By doing so, the chapter enables you to consider applying these six questions to the wide range of information that you will encounter during your mental health nursing programme and throughout your career as a mental health nurse.

Chapter 9 is concerned with critical writing and how you can begin to develop your ability to engage in that form of writing for your university assignments. In particular, it examines what has been referred to as 'the rule of three', which is a way of understanding your critical writing in terms of a three-part structure. Throughout the chapter you are encouraged to think about, and work in accordance with, the rule of three in order to begin to develop your ability to organise and express the content of your critical writing in a systematic, coherent and convincing manner.

Requirements for the NMC *Standards for Pre-registration Nursing Education*

The Nursing and Midwifery Council (NMC) has established standards of competence to be met by applicants to different parts of the register, and these are the standards it considers necessary for safe and effective practice. There are generic standards that all nursing students irrespective of their field must achieve, and field-specific standards relating to each field of nursing, i.e. mental health, children's, learning disability and adult nursing. This book uses those NMC standards, taken from *Standards for Pre-registration Nursing Education* (NMC 2010), to help you understand and meet the competencies required for entry to the NMC register. In particular, the relevant standards of competence are presented at the start of each chapter so that you can clearly see which ones the chapter addresses. While most chapters have generic standards, you will also find that some chapters identify mental health field-specific standards.

Learning features

Throughout the book you will find activities in the text that will help you to make sense of, and learn about, the material being presented by the author.

Some activities ask you to reflect on aspects of practice, or your experience of it, or the people or situations you encounter. *Reflection* is an essential skill in nursing, and it helps you to understand the world around you and often to identify how things might be improved. Other activities will help you develop key skills, such as your ability to *think critically* about a topic in order to challenge received wisdom, or your ability to *research a topic and find appropriate information and evidence,* and to be able to make decisions using that evidence in situations that are often difficult and time-pressured. Finally, communication and working as part of a team are central to all nursing practice, and some activities will ask you to carry out *group activities* or think about your *communication skills* to help develop these.

All the activities require you to take a break from reading the text, think through the issues presented and carry out some independent study, possibly using the internet. Where appropriate, sample answers are presented at the end of each chapter, and these will help you to understand more fully your own reflections and independent study. Remember, academic study will always require independent work; attending lecturers will never be enough to be successful on your programme, and these activities will help to deepen your knowledge and understanding of the issues under scrutiny and give you practice at working on your own.

You might want to think about completing these activities as part of your personal development plan (PDP) or portfolio. After completing the activity, write it up in your PDP or portfolio in a section devoted to that particular skill, then look back over time to see how far you have developed. You can also do more of the activities if you identify a weakness in a key skill, and this will help build your skill and confidence in this area.

There are explanations in the Glossary for words in **bold** in the text.

Chapter 1
Critical thinking

Chapter aims

By the end of this chapter you will be able to:

- define critical thinking;
- identify the benefits that are associated with critical thinking and discuss the significance of critical thinking for mental health nursing;
- describe the primary intellectual skills that are associated with excellence in critical thinking;
- describe the primary emotional attributes that are associated with excellence in critical thinking.

Introduction

There has arguably never been a more exciting time to become a mental health nurse. You are entering a field of health care in which established practices and traditional ways of understanding mental health and distress are being challenged, both by those who work within and those who use contemporary mental health services. The authority of mental health professionals and the legitimacy of their interventions are open to question as never before, and those who use mental health services are increasingly calling for greater involvement in how their experiences are understood and addressed. However, while contemporary mental health nursing is an exciting, dynamic and changing field of health care, it is also a complex and challenging one. The roles that mental health nurses are expected to perform are becoming increasingly sophisticated, and while this brings greater professional **autonomy** and freedom, it also brings with it greater levels of personal **accountability**. As a contemporary mental health nurse you will not only be expected to appreciate the value of theory, research and evidence for your practice, but you will also be expected to identify, evaluate and apply that information actively so that it informs your clinical judgements and decisions. As well as working in an evidence-based manner, you will be expected to work in a collaborative and recovery-focused way with those who use mental health services and this will require an awareness of how your own assumptions, values and beliefs may affect your practice in both productive and non-productive ways. In this changing and challenging environment, you will not only be expected to take responsibility for your own personal and professional development but you will also be required to contribute to, and even take a lead in, the development, implementation and evaluation of mental health services more generally. Contemporary mental health nursing therefore demands that you become an informed, self-aware and proactive mental health practitioner and, central to achieving this, as we shall detail throughout this chapter, is the ability to think critically.

Case study

Jennifer is approaching the end of the first year of her mental health nursing programme and, although she has passed all of her university assignments, she is disappointed that her grades have not been higher. In order to attempt to address this, she has been re-reading the feedback on her assignments from a number of tutors who have consistently identified that her work is 'clear', 'displays evidence of wider reading' and has a 'coherent, logical structure'; however, the feedback also repeatedly suggests that her work is 'largely descriptive' and could be improved by 'demonstrating a greater degree of critical thinking'. While Jennifer is keen to learn from the feedback on her assignments in order to improve her grades, and while she has discussed the feedback with a number of her mental health nursing student colleagues, she remains unsure about what is meant by 'critical thinking'.

The purpose of this chapter is to introduce you to the notion of critical thinking in mental health nursing. In doing so, it will begin by providing a provisional definition of that notion before discussing the significance and the importance of thinking critically for mental health nursing. However, in order to develop and deepen that understanding of critical thinking, this chapter will suggest that it is an activity that is closely associated with a variety of intellectual skills as well as a number of emotional attributes. While a wide variety of intellectual skills have been associated with thinking critically, this chapter will discuss four that are associated with excellence in critical thinking; in particular, it will examine the manner in which thinking critically in mental health nursing requires you to develop your ability to ask questions, to engage in analysis, to develop the capacity to reason and to consider how best to communicate the process and the results of your thinking. Similarly, while a wide variety of emotional attributes have been associated with thinking critically, this chapter will discuss four that are associated with excellence in critical thinking; in particular, it will examine the manner in which thinking critically requires you to develop and maintain a sense of curiosity, to display courage, to develop increasing levels of self-awareness and, finally, to maintain humility and a receptiveness towards alternative perspectives in contemporary mental health care. It is important to recognise that the intellectual skills and emotional attributes associated with critical thinking may take time, practice and patience to develop; however, throughout this chapter you will be encouraged to reflect upon, and work in accordance with, these skills and attributes in order to begin to develop your ability to think critically in mental health nursing.

A definition of critical thinking

Certainly in academic settings, and increasingly in the clinical area, critical thinking is a highly valued activity. You may already have encountered the term during your mental health nursing programme and, like Jennifer in the above case study, you might even have been encouraged or instructed to demonstrate a greater degree of critical thinking in your university assignments. Despite this, it may not have been made clear to you what the term means, let alone how you might begin to develop your ability to think critically. If this is the case, it might be reassuring to know that it is a significant challenge to attempt to convey in words, in a succinct way, the numerous elements and features that comprise an activity as complex as critical thinking. Indeed, critical thinking is a multidimensional **cognitive** and **affective** activity that involves the employment of a wide range of intellectual skills and emotional attributes that are used for a variety of purposes. Of course, definitions have been proposed and it will be productive for you to access, read and carefully consider a number of these (Brookfield 2001; Dewey 2012; Paul & Elder 2014). However, the desire to produce a concise definition of an activity as complex as critical thinking often means that one definition will downplay or even omit elements and features that another emphasises. While they will assist you to begin to understand what is involved in the activity of critical thinking, any definition should perhaps be seen as a provisional formulation that will require further elaboration and consideration. With this in mind, we can suggest that:

> *Critical thinking involves, but is not limited to, the analysis and clarification of issues and areas of concern; the gathering and appraisal of evidence, research and theory; the questioning and challenging of assumptions, values and beliefs; the synthesis and application of information to*

produce alternative and innovative ways of thinking and doing things. To achieve these objectives critical thinkers engage both their intellectual and emotional capabilities in a purposeful, disciplined and often creative manner.

Activity 1.1   *Reflection*

Carefully re-read this definition of critical thinking and highlight any words or phrases that stand out for you as being significant, unusual or unexpected. Try and explain your reasons for why that is.

As this activity is based on your own reflections, there is no outline answer at the end of the chapter.

Critical thinking in mental health nursing

Critical thinking has been identified as delivering a broad range of benefits both to the individual and society more generally. Improvements in concentration and observation, an enhanced ability to gather and evaluate information, greater coherence and clarity in self-expression, more productive and efficient working practices and even the maintenance of a democratic society have all been associated with critical thinking (Brookfield 2001; Cottrell 2011). The importance of facilitating the development of student nurses' critical thinking skills has also been identified as bringing a wide range of benefits to the profession, irrespective of the field of nursing under consideration. Commonly, critical thinking is presented as being central to the appraisal of knowledge and research, and therefore the ability to practise in an evidence-based manner, as well as being associated with a variety of clinical activities such as decision making and judgement, collaborative working and leadership, personal and professional development, the identification of ethically problematic practices and the improvement of services and client care (Price & Harrington 2013; Aveyard *et al.* 2015; Roberts & Ion 2015).

Case study

David and Monique, both second-year mental health nursing students, are discussing their course and, in particular, the emphasis that is placed on being able to think critically. Although David suggests that critical thinking has some value in an academic context, he doesn't see its worth in the clinical area. Indeed, he proposes that mental health nursing is about 'getting things done' and there's no time for critical thinking when the priority should be caring for those who use mental health services.

Monique agrees that mental health nursing is about getting things done but is not so sure that thinking critically is as separate from the provision of mental health care as David seems to think. She has discovered that critical thinking involves questioning what is currently taken for granted and thinking about alternative ways of doing things. Therefore, Monique wonders how mental distress might still be understood, and what practices might still be in existence, if people in the past had not thought critically about the provision of mental health care.

While being fundamental to improving the experiences of those who use mental health services,
the development of your critical thinking capabilities will also be necessary in so far as you are
entering a rapidly changing and often disputed field of health care. Indeed, the basic presuppositions and clinical practices of mental health care are subject to question and challenge unlike
any other area of health care, both by those who work within and those who use mental health
services. Of course, there are questions and disputes in other fields of health care, but these rarely
concern the theoretical foundations, core practices or very existence of the field under consideration. As Bracken and Thomas (2001) suggest, while a number of issues of concern may be raised
in general medicine – such as the length of waiting lists, the quality of practitioners' training and
the adequacy of available resources and equipment – few would question the enterprise or very
existence of medicine itself; indeed, it is difficult to imagine an 'anti-paediatric', 'post-cardiology'
or 'critical anaesthetics' movement, yet the so-called 'anti-psychiatry' movement and, more
recently, the 'post' or 'critical-psychiatry' movement illustrates how critical thinking has been, and
continues to be, a characteristic feature of psychiatry and mental health care more generally.
Throughout your training as a mental health nursing student, it will therefore be important for
you not only to become aware of, but also to become responsive to, the questions, debates and
issues of concern that characterise contemporary mental health care and this will demand that
you develop your critical thinking capabilities. Rather than simply following instruction and performing tasks without significant understanding and evaluation, you will be required as never
before to appraise and justify the information, evidence and knowledge which informs the whole
range of your clinical work. As such, it will be necessary for you to develop the ability to question,
challenge and potentially change approaches to mental health care that do not withstand critical
examination, especially in response to contemporary research and evidence, the emergence of
new theoretical approaches or because of the active involvement and innovative work of those
who use mental health services.

Critical thinking and intellectual skills

So far we have presented a provisional definition of critical thinking and considered why thinking critically is important for you as a student of mental health nursing; however, we can now
begin to develop and deepen our understanding of critical thinking further by examining the
particular skills and attributes that are often associated with that activity. In the definition presented above, it was suggested that critical thinking has both cognitive and affective dimensions,
which means that it requires not only the employment of certain intellectual skills but also the

possession of a number of emotional attributes or personal qualities. While a variety of intellectual skills have been associated with excellence in critical thinking – such as interpretation, inference, evaluation, explanation and categorising (Paul & Elder 2014) – the following four are particularly significant for critical thinking in mental health nursing: questioning, analysing, reasoning and communicating.

Questioning

One of the most profound intellectual skills required for thinking critically is the ability to ask questions and to ask searching, significant and important questions in particular. Although the ability to ask questions may seem commonplace, there can be a variety of reasons why you might refrain from doing so.

Case study

Rashida is in the second week of her first clinical placement on an acute mental health ward and, although she has found it challenging and fast-paced at times, she is enjoying the opportunity to gain clinical experience in a mental health care setting. Indeed, Rashida's mentor has already commented on how well she has adapted to the environment and how quickly she appears to have integrated herself into the team. However, while Rashida is beginning to develop her knowledge of the different forms of mental distress that those who use mental health services experience, she has heard some members of staff suggesting that a number of service users have 'behavioural issues' and that some of that behaviour is 'attention seeking'. This is the first time that she has encountered these phrases and she has some concerns and questions about their use; however, she is reluctant to raise them because she doesn't want to be seen as lacking in knowledge or as wasting staff time with what might be viewed as 'silly' or 'unhelpful' questions.

Although there may be multiple reasons why you might not do so, asking questions in mental health nursing is central to the ongoing process of evaluating and improving the experiences of those who use mental health services. However, what questions should you ask and how can you ensure that they are searching, significant and important questions? Perhaps unsurprisingly, the answer to this is complex and a key reason for this complexity is that critical thinkers are often able to perceive problems in mental health care, and raise questions about that care, which other people, for a variety of reasons, do not. This means that critical thinkers often raise questions that others do not initially recognise as important, and even raise questions that others sometimes fail to recognise as valid or meaningful. A central aspect of asking questions is therefore the ability to consider why a question might be important and to be able to respond when people may initially dismiss the question as having an obvious or self-evident answer. Indeed, rather than providing answers, it can be a significant achievement of critical thinking to raise a question that others had not considered or, if they had considered it, thought that the answer to the question was obvious or self-evident. Such questions can enable people to see issues of concern where there was previously thought to be none and can stimulate further investigation, research and, ultimately, different ways of thinking and doing things in contemporary mental health care.

Analysing

In addition to asking questions, and being able to explain why those questions might be worth considering, critical thinkers engage in analysis. Although you may have already encountered the word analysis, and even been instructed to analyse or critically analyse something connected with your mental health nursing programme, the word – like many of the words and phrases associated with critical thinking – can appear complex and difficult to define. In order to begin to understand what analysis means, however, it is instructive to recognise that its literal meaning is 'to loosen' or 'to take things apart'. Analysis can therefore be understood as examining something, which can be anything from a concept to a clinical procedure, in order to attempt to determine its constituent parts or the manner in which it is put together. However, it is sometimes not immediately obvious how something is put together or how something works because many of the practices and knowledge claims in mental health nursing are not only complex but also made up of elements that are often implicit or hidden. Therefore, an important aspect of analysis is not only identifying the relevant parts of something but also 'unearthing' and making explicit the variety of assumptions, values and beliefs that underlie a particular practice or knowledge claim.

Activity 1.3   *Critical thinking*

You may be aware that recovery is an important and prevalent notion in contemporary mental health care and the importance of practising in a recovery-oriented manner may already have been impressed upon you. However, you may not have been given the opportunity to think critically about and analyse the notion of recovery in order to determine the assumptions, values and beliefs that underlie that concept. For this activity, analyse the concept of recovery by considering the following critical questions:

- When understood in the context of contemporary mental health care, does recovery mean that a person no longer has 'signs or symptoms' of mental distress and is 'cured'?
- Is it possible for every person who uses mental health services to recover, irrespective of the particular form of mental distress that s/he is experiencing?
- Are there commonalities between people's experiences of recovery or is it, as is often suggested, a uniquely individual 'journey'?

As this activity is based on your own critical thinking, there is no outline answer at the end of the chapter.

Your responses to these and other analytical questions about recovery will help you to clarify and make explicit many of the assumptions, values and beliefs underlying the use of that concept in contemporary mental health care. However, they will also profoundly influence how you understand the varied forms of mental distress that those who use mental health services experience, as well as determining what you consider to be the most appropriate and beneficial interventions to employ in responding to that distress.

Reasoning

Over the duration of your mental health nursing programme, and over the subsequent course of your career as a mental health nurse, a fundamental critical thinking skill that you will be required to develop will be your ability to reason. At its most fundamental level, reasoning has been presented as identifying and evaluating the reasons given for something, whether that involves the reasons given for doing something in a particular way or the reasons given for understanding something in a particular way (Cottrell 2011). However, the reasons given might not always be explicit and, as a critical thinker, you may even suspect that there are reasons other than the ones stated. In addition, there may be multiple reasons given for why you should understand or be doing things in a particular way and the 'line' or 'chain' of reasoning may be long and complex. For example, the reasons given for understanding or doing something in a particular way might include formal or logical arguments, established or new research, theoretical frameworks or philosophies, financial pressures or resource limitations, previous experience or intuition and even because 'that's the way it's always been done'.

Case study

Michael was admitted to an acute mental health ward earlier today following a rapid deterioration in his mood. Although he has a history of depression, this is his first admission to hospital for a number of years and he is apprehensive about being there. At dinner time he asks if he can eat in his room but is told by a member of staff that he must come to the dining room and eat with the other mental health service users. When he questions the reason for this, he is told that it is 'ward policy'.

One of the primary aims of reasoning is not only to determine what specific reasons are being offered for understanding or doing something in a particular way but also to judge the worth or the merits of those reasons – to judge, for example, whether the response of 'ward policy' in the above case study is a shorthand response beneath which there are valid reasons why people are not permitted to eat in their rooms or whether it is a response that seeks to give credibility to a practice which has no clearly articulated or justifiable reasons. However, while it involves evaluating the reasons of others, a significant component of reasoning is the ability to develop, clarify and articulate your own reasons. If you think that the reasons given for doing or understanding something in contemporary mental health care are not justified, or if you think that things should be done or understood in a different way, then you will need to articulate the reasons for why you think that is the case and you will need to make your reasons robust enough to withstand the questioning, analysis and reasoning of others.

Communicating

When considering the variety of skills that are associated with critical thinking, one of those that is often underestimated is the ability to engage in effective communication. While a variety of reasons for this could be proposed, an enduring reason may be that critical thinking has traditionally been understood as an individual activity. The popular image of the 'deep thinker' is an individual who retreats from the 'hustle and bustle' of everyday life to a place of solitude in order to contemplate seemingly 'profound' or 'lofty' thoughts; however, there is an alternative tradition that understands critical thinking as an activity that occurs between people and is conducted in the midst of the 'noise' of everyday life (Miller 2013). As a mental health nursing student, your critical thinking will be conducted individually and in discussion with others and it may be necessary to communicate both the process and the results of your critical thinking in a variety of written and verbal forms, including essays, exams, presentations and group debates. A fundamental reason for engaging in critical thinking as a mental health nursing student, and certainly as a mental health nurse, is to question, challenge and even consider changing contemporary understandings and practices in mental health care in order to improve the experiences of those who use mental health services. While it is sometimes thought that the sheer quality of a person's critical thinking guarantees that it will be received well by others, as a mental health nursing student you should be starting to appreciate the complex character of interpersonal communication and, in particular, the variety of factors that can inhibit or facilitate effective communication (Walker 2014). In order to improve the chances of your critical thinking being received well – whether by your tutors, your peers, other mental health professionals or by those who use mental health services – you will need to reflect on the whole range of verbal and written communication skills that you are currently developing and consider how they can be best employed to convey your critical thinking to others.

Critical thinking and emotional attributes

While critical thinking is commonly characterised as a purely logical or intellectual activity, throughout this chapter it has been suggested that thinking critically not only requires the employment of intellectual skills but also the possession of a number of emotional attributes or personal qualities. While a variety of these emotional attributes, personal qualities or 'habits of mind' have been associated with excellence in critical thinking – such as integrity, confidence, honesty and self-directedness (Paul & Elder 2014) – the following four are particularly significant for critical thinking in mental health nursing: curiosity, courage, self-awareness and humility.

Curiosity

One of the defining attributes of those who think critically is curiosity. Critical thinkers are characteristically curious, inquisitive people who do not simply accept established norms, values and practices but, at least periodically, wonder why things are the way they are. Critical thinkers in mental health nursing are curious about why it is that we currently understand and do things in a particular way as opposed to other ways and, being so disposed, they are prompted to ask questions and to consider the responses to these questions.

Activity 1.4   *Reflection*

Mental health nursing students are characteristically curious about the field of health care that they are entering and commonly have many interesting questions. Identify one thing about mental health care that you are curious about and present it to your colleagues in the form of a question.

As this activity is based on your own reflections, there is no outline answer at the end of the chapter.

Irrespective of how developed your intellectual skills are, the ability to ask important questions and to engage in analysis and reasoning will be of limited value without the curiosity and inquisitiveness that dispose you to begin asking questions and thinking critically in the first place. However, many mental health nursing students – as they enter the profession and are exposed to new environments, new knowledge claims and new ways of understanding and responding to mental distress – are characteristically curious about many aspects of contemporary mental health care. Therefore, in seeking to develop your critical thinking capabilities, the challenge may not be in developing curiosity as an emotional attribute but rather maintaining that curiosity and inquisitiveness as you progress through your mental health nursing programme and your mental health nursing career. There may be a variety of personal, social and institutional reasons why you might begin to lose curiosity about your chosen field of health care and we shall examine these, along with other impediments to critical thinking, in Chapter 3. For now you should recognise the importance of cultivating curiosity in order to develop your critical thinking capabilities and, at least periodically, pause to look at your own practice and the practice of those around you in order to question why it is that we currently understand and do things the way that we do.

Courage

As well as possessing and maintaining curiosity about the way things are, a key emotional attribute that is necessary for critical thinking is courage. It may not be immediately obvious why critical thinking requires courage until you remember that a central aspect of thinking critically involves asking questions about our own assumptions, values and beliefs. To subject one's own presuppositions to this degree of critical examination can be profoundly anxiety provoking and we ought not to underestimate how attached we can become to our own way of understanding and doing things. Indeed, Brookfield (2001, p. 7) suggests that *We may well feel fearful of the consequences that might arise from contemplating alternatives to our current ways of thinking and living; resistance, resentment, and confusion are evident at various stages in the critical thinking process.* Critical thinking in mental health nursing, however, can involve not only calling into question our own ways of understanding and doing things but also questioning, analysing and reasoning about how other individuals, other groups, whole disciplines or even entire organisations understand and do things. Similar to the variety of reasons why we may be reluctant to question our knowledge and practices, there may be a variety of reasons why other individuals, groups, disciplines and organisations are reluctant to question their knowledge, procedures and protocols. To engage in critical thinking in the context of a busy mental health care environment where there is often a strong emphasis on getting things done may be regarded as a distraction or annoyance at best and, at worst, as a dangerous and subversive challenge to the efficient functioning of the team within which you work. Critical thinking will therefore require you to display courage to ask questions when such activity can potentially rouse a variety of challenging responses; similarly, it will also require you to display resilience and perseverance in order to continue to engage in that activity when faced with the possibility of individual and collective resistance and resentment.

Self-awareness

As we have already noted, critical thinkers ask questions, engage in analysis and reason about a variety of things, including their own assumptions, values and beliefs. As a consequence, they not only become increasingly aware of their own values and beliefs, but they also become aware of the potential to form powerful and often biased emotional attachments to their own way of understanding and doing things; therefore, in developing their self-awareness, critical thinkers also seek to manage that emotional attachment.

Case study

Although Emily has decided that she would like to pursue a career in mental health nursing, she has strong feelings about the use of electroconvulsive therapy (ECT). She has seen images of its use in films and on the internet and has read that it can cause memory loss and maybe even permanent damage to the brain. How can it still be justified to pass electricity through someone's brain in order to treat mental distress, especially when no one knows how it works? Emily thinks that this intervention is 'barbaric' and passionately believes that it should have no place in contemporary mental health care.

Critical thinking is sometimes characterised as a dispassionate, detached activity that opposes the influence of the emotions such that, in order to think critically, it is considered necessary to 'put aside' those emotions in order to maintain the strictest standards of 'pure' rationality and critical thought. However, critical thinkers are aware that emotional engagement with an issue, such as that displayed by Emily in the above case study, can be a powerful and productive force for thinking critically. It can not only direct but also sustain continued critical debate, investigation and research into the legitimacy of interventions that many people oppose, such as ECT. However, those who think critically are also aware that opposition based solely on anger, outrage or incredulity, no matter how intensely those emotions are felt, is insufficient; rather, such emotional conviction will need to be accompanied by informed analysis, argument and reasons before it can be considered an instance of critical thinking. Moreover, the emotional self-awareness and management that are associated with those who seek to develop their capacity to think critically do not mean that critical thinkers somehow have control or mastery over their emotions. Indeed, while critical thinkers display an awareness of the power of the emotions both as a productive and non-productive influence upon their thinking, they are continually seeking to develop the ability to harness the productive influence and diminish the non-productive influence.

15

Humility

Critical thinkers are sometimes characterised as critical people. In particular, they are presented as judgemental people who are concerned with criticising and finding fault with the efforts of others and who do so from a position of supposed superiority without making any positive contributions themselves. However, while critical thinking can involve evaluating and making judgements about the relative merits of various assumptions, beliefs and arguments, there is nothing inherently negative about thinking critically. Indeed, rather than superiority or fault finding, a quality that is often associated with excellence in critical thinking is humility. As critical thinkers continue to ask questions, and analyse and reason about the responses to those questions, they increasingly become aware that there are multiple ways of understanding and doing things; other societies, other cultures and other historical periods have understood things in ways that are sometimes very different from our own. Critical thinkers in mental health nursing are aware that there are diverse approaches to mental health and distress and that our current understandings and practices are profoundly influenced by our particular social, cultural and historical perspectives. While we may think that our current approach to mental health and distress is sophisticated, productive and superior to previous approaches, critical thinkers are aware that it is not final and definitive. As previous approaches to mental health care have changed as a consequence of various social, cultural and historical forces, critical thinkers display humility in their awareness that our current understandings and practices will change as a consequence of similar forces. Of course, such an awareness of the diverse approaches to mental health and distress does not mean that critical thinkers are ready to accept the latest perspective or that all perspectives are equally valid. Critical thinkers are characteristically sceptical of the uncritical acceptance of the latest perspectives and the 'buzz' words and phrases that often accompany them, and they are equally sceptical of those who claim to have arrived at final, definitive explanations about mental health and distress. Rather, the humility that is associated with an awareness of the provisional character of our current understandings and practices in contemporary mental health care entails a receptiveness to new ideas from a variety of sources and a willingness to subject them to the questioning, analysis and reasoning that characterise critical thinking.

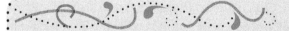

Chapter summary

In this chapter we have discussed the notion of critical thinking and the significance of thinking critically in the rapidly changing and often disputed field of contemporary mental health care. While critical thinking is to be understood as a complex, challenging and multidimensional activity, we have provided a provisional definition of what that activity involves and suggested that it is associated with a variety of intellectual skills as well as a number of emotional attributes. In particular, critical thinking in mental health nursing requires you to develop your ability to ask questions, to engage in analysis, to develop the capacity to reason and to consider how best to communicate the process and the results of your thinking. In addition, it has been suggested that critical thinking requires you to maintain curiosity about current approaches to mental health and distress, to display

continued . . .

self-awareness and courage towards the resistance that this can create as well as developing humility and a receptiveness towards alternative approaches to, and perspectives on, contemporary mental health care. As with any skill or attribute, those associated with critical thinking will take time to develop and will need to be practised regularly; however, this chapter has encouraged you to begin to reflect upon, and work in accordance with, those skills and attributes in order to develop your ability to think critically in mental health nursing and thereby move towards becoming an informed, proactive and critically engaged mental health professional.

Activities: brief outline answers

Activity 1.2 Team working

There are a number of comprehensive, stimulating and controversial accounts of how mental distress has historically been understood and it will be productive to access and consider such accounts (Shorter 1997; Foucault 2001; Porter 2003; Scull 2011, 2015). However, when thinking about the historical origins of contemporary mental health care – and how that which is now variously referred to as mental illness, disorder or distress has been understood in the past – it is important to be cautious about thinking of such history in simplistic terms as a continuous, progressive movement from less sophisticated to more advanced understandings and interventions. Indeed, multiple and competing histories have been written that illustrate how different understandings and responses to mental distress sought to gain dominance at different times, with it being far from obvious which would prevail. However, in your discussions with your colleagues, you may have identified, for instance, that mental distress has been understood in the past in overtly religious terms, in terms of the soul's possession by spirits and demons or as the result of God's vengeance for moral failings, and that a variety of spiritual means were employed to respond to such a condition, including prayer, pilgrimage or exorcism. You may also have noted that, while mental distress has been understood in the past as possessing its own wisdom, during the seventeenth and eighteenth centuries it increasingly began to be thought of as the result of a problem of thinking, of irrationality, for which a variety of treatments were used to 'shock' a person back to rationality, such as whirling chairs and 'baths of surprise'. Finally, you may have also discussed the confinement of people in a variety of institutions, including private for-profit 'madhouses' and public 'lunatic asylums'. The quality of care received in such institutions varied widely depending on a person's wealth, social status and family network but, for the poor, life inside such institutions could be harsh; for example, you may have discussed how a person inside such an institution could be subject to various forms of physical restraint, such as the use of chains, belts and straitjackets and multiple invasive treatments such as purges, vomits and blood letting.

Further reading

Brookfield SD (2001) *Developing Critical Thinkers: Challenging adults to explore alternative ways of thinking and acting.* Milton Keynes: Open University Press.

This is a stimulating book that discusses a variety of strategies that can be employed for facilitating critical thinking in adults and how to assist adults to do so in different areas of their life.

Cottrell S (2011) *Critical Thinking Skills: Developing effective analysis and argument*, 2nd edition. Basingstoke: Palgrave Macmillan.

Although not specific to health care, this book provides a comprehensive account of how to develop a range of critical thinking skills such as the evaluation of arguments, the identification of assumptions and the appraisal of evidence.

Paul R & Elder L (2014) *Critical Thinking: Tools for taking charge of your professional and personal life,* 2nd edition. Upper Saddle River, NJ: Pearson Education.

This is a comprehensive and detailed work that discusses many aspects of critical thinking and provides, among other things, an informative discussion about the emotional attributes or personal qualities that are associated with critical thinking.

Price B & Harrington A (2013) *Critical Thinking and Writing for Nursing Students,* 2nd edition. London: Sage/Learning Matters.

This book provides an accessible introduction to critical thinking and writing for nursing students, and includes numerous activities to assist in the development of these skills in the context of contemporary nursing theory and practice.

Useful websites

www.criticalpsychiatry.co.uk

This is the website for the Critical Psychiatry Network, where you will find resources and articles produced by a variety of people who employ critical thinking to question, analyse and reason about many aspects of contemporary mental health care.

www.criticalthinking.org

Here you will find the website for the Centre for Critical Thinking, which provides a variety of resources and information on critical thinking, including how its development can be facilitated in educational settings and throughout society more generally.

Chapter 2
Critical reflection

Chapter aims

By the end of this chapter you will be able to:

- define critical reflection;
- identify the benefits that are associated with critical reflection and discuss the significance of critical reflection for mental health nursing;
- describe the underlying principles and key stages associated with critical reflection;
- apply the stages of critical reflection to your own clinical experiences in mental health nursing.

Introduction

Case study

Richard completed his first mental health nursing examination earlier today and, as he waits for the train home, he is becoming increasingly concerned that it may not have gone particularly well. While he thinks that his answer to the question on depression was fairly comprehensive, he was not expecting such a difficult question about the arguments for the biological basis of schizophrenia. Perhaps he should have started to revise earlier, but this semester has been extremely busy and he has struggled to balance his clinical placements, university assignments and everything else that has been happening at home. However, he is resolved to manage his time more effectively and to be better prepared for his future university assignments; therefore, he begins to wonder if from now on he should spend a couple of evenings a week in the library reviewing and revising the large amount of information that is being introduced during his mental health nursing programme.

You will almost certainly have already engaged in reflection at some point and perhaps even in a manner similar to Richard's reflections in the above case study. In its everyday sense, reflection refers to the contemplation of something, often an event or an experience, and it is an activity that you might have engaged in for a variety of reasons. For example, you might have reflected on an event or an experience in order to try and clarify what happened and why it happened in the particular way that it did, and you might also have reflected on that event or experience in order to try and learn something from it and ensure that whatever happened does not happen again. Like Richard, it may be that you reflect when you are on your own and when you have a moment to yourself or it may be that you engage in reflection by talking things through with others. Sometimes you may reflect on a recent event that strikes you as particularly important – and you may even have noticed that you are able to reflect in the middle of events as they occur – while at other times you may reflect on events that happened weeks, months or even years ago. Those events may be ones in which you were intimately involved, and they may have been happy or particularly unpleasant experiences, or you may have reflected on events or experiences that happened to others and which seem only indirectly related to you. Indeed, it has been suggested that reflection is such a common, everyday human activity that to live a life without reflecting upon and examining the variety of events and experiences that make up our lives would not only be out of the ordinary but may even be unfeasible (Rolfe *et al.* 2011). Over the last several decades, however, the activity of reflection has gained increased attention in both academic and clinical environments and, while having commonalities with such everyday reflection, has come to denote a more rigorous and systematic activity. A variety of conceptual models and frameworks have been devised to attempt to clarify what the process of reflection involves, while a number of techniques, methods and strategies have been introduced to provide guidance on how best to engage in reflection. Similarly, the purpose of reflection has been formulated in a number of ways, with it variously being suggested that its value resides in being an activity to improve clinical practice, to direct health care research, to facilitate the learning of practitioners and to improve the experiences of those who use health care services (Jasper 2003; Taylor 2010; Bulman & Schutz 2013).

The purpose of this chapter is to introduce you to the notion of critical reflection in mental health nursing. A variety of terms are used in the literature when discussing reflection, such as 'reflective practice', 'reflective learning' and 'critical reflection'; sometimes these terms are used interchangeably and sometimes differences are drawn between them. In this chapter, we shall be using the term critical reflection and over the course of the chapter we shall distinguish that term by highlighting the critical aspect of reflection and, in particular, its relationship to the activity of critical thinking. In doing so, a provisional definition of critical reflection is provided before highlighting the benefits of that activity and discussing its significance for you as a mental health nursing student and, subsequently, as a mental health nurse. While a variety of models and frameworks have been devised in order to help clarify what the process of reflection involves, we shall highlight three underlying principles and key stages that will help you to understand and engage in the activity of critical reflection. However, over the course of your studies as a mental health nursing student, and over the course of your career as a mental health nurse, there will be an expectation that you will engage in the activity of critical reflection for a variety of reasons, including your continuing personal and professional development. Therefore, this chapter will encourage you to begin to apply critical reflection to your clinical experiences and, in doing so, assist you in beginning to move towards becoming a critically reflective practitioner in contemporary mental health nursing.

A definition of critical reflection

It is common for mental health nursing students to be introduced to the notion of reflection early on in their studies and you may already have been instructed to reflect on a learning experience at university or in the clinical area. However, as with critical thinking, what reflection means, or how you might go about engaging in the reflective process, may not have been made particularly clear to you. There may be multiple reasons for this but it has been suggested that the very popularity of the notion of reflection has meant that its meaning is often assumed to be obvious and therefore defining reflection is often overlooked and even seen as unnecessary (White *et al.* 2006). Similarly, the contemporary popularity of reflection has meant that the term is often simply 'tagged' on to a variety of activities in an attempt to add credibility to them while, as indicated above, terms associated with reflection are referred to without it being particularly clear how they are being used. Indeed, it has been suggested that the term reflection is being so indiscriminately used that it is rapidly becoming a 'catch-all' term that is coming to mean all things to all people (Rolfe *et al.* 2011). Despite this, there are notable attempts to provide a rigorous definition of reflection and you should access, read and consider these carefully (Boyd & Fales 1983; Boud *et al.* 1985; Dewey 2012). However, while it should be remembered that reflection is a complex, multi-dimensional concept, and while you should perhaps treat any definition of reflection as provisional and in need of further elaboration and consideration, we can suggest that:

Critical reflection is that activity in which experiences are considered in order to identify the assumptions influencing the thoughts, feelings and actions in a given situation. These assumptions are then rigorously questioned and challenged with a view to developing alternative ways of thinking, feeling and acting in future situations.

This definition makes it clear that the ability to identify assumptions is a central feature of critical reflection. Assumptions can be ideas, values and beliefs that we assume to be the case, commonly held without evidence or good reason, and that influence our thoughts, feelings and actions, often without us being aware that they are doing so. We all inherit a wide range of assumptions from a variety of sources and, while those assumptions can help us prepare for, and make sense of, events and experiences, some of our assumptions may be questionable, misinformed or even simply wrong.

For this activity, think back to a time before you became a mental health nursing student and attempt to identify your assumptions about people who were given a diagnosis of schizophrenia.

- What did you assume were the possible causes of schizophrenia?
- Did you assume that people with a diagnosis of schizophrenia would behave in certain ways?
- What did you assume was the treatment for those with a diagnosis of schizophrenia?
- Were your assumptions about schizophrenia correct or, in retrospect, do you think they were questionable, misinformed or even simply wrong?

As this activity is based on your own reflections, there is no outline answer at the end of the chapter.

Critical reflection in mental health nursing

The notion of critical reflection can be understood as having origins that date back at least to ancient Greece. Indeed, the Athenian philosopher Socrates not only stressed the importance of reflecting and critically examining one's assumptions, values and beliefs, but also famously suggested that the unexamined life was a life not worth living (Plato 1961). However, most of the contemporary literature acknowledges the importance of John Dewey (1997) and Donald Schön (1983) as being influential in the resurgence of interest in reflection and its significance for the development of the acquisition and employment of knowledge for professional practice. Indeed, Schön (1983) is often referred to in the literature for introducing an important distinction that you should be aware of between **reflection-in-action** and **reflection-on-action**.

Concept summary: Reflection-in-action and reflection-on-action

Reflection-in-action refers to the process by which practitioners think about an aspect of their clinical work while in the midst of doing it. This is sometimes referred to as 'thinking on our feet', in which practitioners adapt their clinical performance from moment to moment depending on the demands of the situation.

Reflection-on-action refers to the activity in which practitioners think about an aspect of their clinical work after the event has occurred. Doing so provides the practitioner with the opportunity to spend more time thinking about what has occurred in a rigorous, systematic and considered manner.

Much of the health care literature on reflection has been concerned with exploring and developing Schön's notion of reflection-on-action. The participation of nurses in reflection-on-action, and reflecting on their clinical experiences and practice in particular, has been associated with a broad range of benefits for the individual practitioner, for those who use health care services, for health care organisations and for nursing as a profession. In particular, structured, systematic and considered reflection has variously been suggested to help practitioners identify gaps in their knowledge, skills and experience; to avoid routine practice and promote **evidence-based practice**; to increase the self-awareness and confidence of practitioners; to ensure better standards of patient safety and a reduction in adverse incidents; to improve clinical supervision arrangements and training opportunities and to encourage the development of nursing's knowledge base and a recognition of its unique contribution to client care (Jasper 2006; Howatson-Jones 2013; Bolton 2014).

While acknowledging the broad range of benefits associated with reflection, however, it is important to recognise that critical reflection will be particularly valuable for you as a mental health nursing student and, subsequently, throughout your career as a mental health nurse. In order to understand why this is the case, you should remember that a central characteristic of critical reflection is the ability to identify and rigorously challenge the assumptions, both your own and those of others, that influence the range of thoughts, feelings and actions that are present in a given situation. Indeed, the critical element in critical reflection is the ability to employ the range of intellectual skills and emotional attributes associated with critical thinking and apply them to the wide range of events and experiences that occur throughout all aspects of contemporary mental health care. Critical reflection will therefore require you to analyse and 'unearth' the assumptions that are influencing a particular situation, to ask searching and challenging questions about those assumptions and to evaluate whether there are good reasons for holding those assumptions or whether alternative perspectives ought to be considered.

Case study

Two mental health nurses, Caitlin and William, are reflecting together on the recent suicide attempt by a mental health service user on the ward. As they do so, Caitlin says that she was very surprised by the incident because the service user had been talking about suicide and self-harm beforehand and that is often an indication that a person will not act upon such stated intentions. William agrees that people who are serious about suicide do not talk about it. He adds that, as mental health nurses, they are in an extremely difficult position because if they talk to those who use mental health services about suicide and self-harm behaviours then this will encourage them to think about this more and they are then more likely to act upon those thoughts. Caitlin agrees that they have a very difficult job and concludes by stating that if a person is serious about committing suicide then, ultimately, there is very little that they can do to prevent it.

> **Activity 2.2**   *Critical thinking*
>
> In their joint reflection Caitlin and William are beginning to express and make explicit their assumptions about suicide and self-harm.
>
> - What are those assumptions?
> - Do you think those assumptions are correct?
> - What might be the consequences of not critically reflecting upon, and thinking critically about, those assumptions?
>
> *An outline answer is provided at the end of the chapter.*

As the joint reflection by Caitlin and William in the above case study illustrates, the activity of reflection can occur without that reflection possessing a critical element. It is possible to reflect in such a manner that the assumptions that are influencing a particular situation are not identified or, if they are identified, are not subject to rigorous questioning and critical examination. Indeed, it has been suggested that reflective activities that do not employ critical thinking could potentially perpetuate or produce poor practice and may even maintain or lead to dangerous practice (Thompson & Thompson 2008). Therefore, in order to provide informed, responsive and safe mental health care it will be necessary for you to develop your critical thinking capabilities so that you are able to bring this critical element to your reflective activity. To the extent that your assumptions can profoundly influence, in both productive and non-productive ways, how you understand and respond to a person's mental distress then it will be necessary for you to identify, challenge and potentially change your assumptions, especially in response to contemporary research and evidence, the emergence of new theoretical approaches or because of the active involvement and innovative work of those who use mental health services.

The stages of critical reflection

In order to provide rigour and structure to the process of reflection, a variety of reflective models and frameworks have been devised. Some commonly used models and frameworks include those proposed by Borton (1970), Kolb (1984), Gibbs (1988) and Johns (2004), while models and frameworks of reflection that possess an explicitly critical element include those devised by Kim (1999) and Taylor (2010). There is no obligation for you to use a model or framework but they can be useful, particularly when first beginning to critically reflect, in helping to provide a degree of structure and coherence to the process. Over time, however, you may find that you develop your own particular manner of reflecting critically, and it will be worthwhile accessing and testing out a number of models and frameworks in order to see which suits your particular way of engaging in critical reflection. Despite the diversity of models and frameworks, however, Jasper (2003) has noted that reflection involves three basic components: experience, reflection and action. As illustrated in Figure 2.1, these three components can be presented as three stages in a reflective cycle, what Jasper (2003) refers to as the ERA cycle, and they can assist you to begin to think about, and practically engage in, the process of critical reflection in mental health nursing.

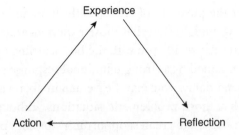

Figure 2.1: Jasper's (2003) experience–reflection–action (ERA) cycle.

Experience

Case study

Philippa is a newly appointed community mental health nurse who has recently begun to visit Leon after he was discharged from hospital. Now in his early 30s, Leon first became involved with mental health services in his early 20s while at university, when he began to experience auditory hallucinations. He was given a diagnosis of schizophrenia and has since had numerous admissions to hospital, with the most recent coinciding with the breakdown of his relationship with his long-term partner. As a newly appointed community mental health nurse, Philippa is understandably a little apprehensive about her new role and her meetings with Leon are beginning to cause her concern. In reflecting upon these meetings she notes that Leon talks at length about his 'voices', particularly about those he finds distressing, and she thinks that his 'preoccupation' with them may be an indication that his mental health is deteriorating. She vaguely remembers learning somewhere about the importance of not 'reinforcing' auditory hallucinations and has attempted to discuss and employ a variety of distraction techniques with Leon. She has also provided him with information about his diagnosis and has attempted to explain that his auditory hallucinations are a symptom of that mental health problem. However, she is disappointed that none of her interventions seem to have been received particularly well by Leon and she is now considering the possibility of discussing a review of his medication with the medical team.

To be able to engage in the process of critical reflection then, like Philippa in the above case study, it will be necessary for you to identify an experience upon which to reflect. However, for critical reflection to be a meaningful activity, the experience that you choose ought to be one that not only possesses some significance for you but also provides you with an opportunity to develop an aspect of your professional practice. This may be a particular challenge when you first begin to reflect critically because, as a mental health nursing student, you will have a wide range of clinical experiences to draw upon, and you may be unsure how to go about selecting an experience that provides you with the best learning opportunity. To a certain extent, selecting an experience may initially be a matter of 'trial and error' and one that you will become more skilled at the more you engage in the reflective process. However, to help you select from your range of clinical experiences it can be useful to consider those that somehow seemed problematic to you. Of course, reflecting upon positive experiences can also be productive but, for the purposes of critical reflection, and critically examining your assumptions in particular, you might find that those experiences in which things did not go as well as you had expected will provide you with the best learning opportunities. Such experiences can often be accompanied by a strong emotional response such as frustration or disappointment and, understandably, you may be reluctant to revisit them. However, it is important to recognise that those problematic situations, although perhaps emotionally uncomfortable, can often possess the greatest opportunity for both personal and professional development if you are able to respond to them in productive ways.

Activity 2.3   *Reflection*

From the range of clinical experiences that you have had so far as a mental health nursing student, choose one that you think will provide you with the best opportunity to engage in critical reflection. In order to help you decide, remember that an experience in which things did not go as well as you had hoped might enable you to get the most out of the process of critical reflection.

As this activity is based on your own reflections, there is no outline answer at the end of the chapter.

As well as identifying an experience that will provide you with a significant learning opportunity, critical reflection requires you to attempt to get clear about what happened in that situation. This will mean that your reflections at this stage are largely descriptive as you attempt both to determine what were the key features of the experience and also formulate what the particular problem or issue of concern was. As this is your reflection, then you may understandably be giving an account of the experience from your own perspective and, of course, it is essential that you do so. However, you may find that you are able to give a fuller, more balanced account of the experience if you attempt to do so not only from your own perspective but also from the perspective of others. Rather than only describing what your actions, thoughts and feelings were in the situation, you can also attempt to provide an account of the thoughts, feelings and actions of others who may have been involved in the situation, such as your peers, qualified members of staff and, importantly, those who use mental health services. This will not only give you a broader, more balanced account of the experience but may also assist you in clarifying its key features and issues of concern, and therefore enable you to obtain greater insights into the experience – insights that a description from your perspective alone may not have produced.

Activity 2.4   *Reflection*

Having chosen an experience upon which to reflect, attempt to provide a detailed and balanced description of that experience by asking yourself, and responding to, a series of exploratory questions. In developing Borton's (1970) reflective framework, Rolfe (2011) has proposed the following cue questions that might help you:

continued . . .

- What was the problem or issue of concern in this experience?
- What was my role in the situation?
- What was I trying to achieve?
- What actions did I take?
- What was the response of others?
- What have been the consequences for the service user, for myself and for others?
- What thoughts and feelings did it invoke in the service user, in myself and in others?
- What was good and what was bad about the experience?

As this activity is based on your own reflections, there is no outline answer at the end of the chapter.

Reflection

Case study

In beginning to reflect critically upon the assumptions underlying her experience, Philippa considers the knowledge, values and beliefs that are informing her clinical assessment, decisions and interventions with Leon. She is confident that the information that she has been giving him about schizophrenia and auditory hallucinations is recognised as being well established. However, she is less confident about the grounds for her belief that auditory hallucinations ought not to be discussed with Leon because this will result in them being reinforced. Similarly, after a brief internet search and discussion with a colleague, she is unsure about the effectiveness of distraction techniques as a long-term strategy for dealing with auditory hallucinations. Indeed, she is discovering that there are some organisations who promote an alternative perspective on auditory hallucinations that differs significantly from that maintained by traditional psychiatry. Rather than understanding them as a by-product or meaningless symptom of a mental health problem, this perspective understands auditory hallucinations – or what it refers to as 'hearing voices' – as a meaningful experience that is often related to unresolved and often distressing events in a person's life. It therefore seeks to discuss the voice-hearing experience with a view to helping develop 'frameworks of understanding' that enable a person to make sense of, and cope with, that experience in the context of that person's unique life history.

Having identified an experience that you think may provide you with a significant learning opportunity, and having given a balanced description of it, the next stage of the ERA cycle requires you to reflect critically upon that experience. If the previous stage required your reflections to be largely descriptive and to give an account of that experience in terms of what happened then, like Philippa in the above case study, this stage requires you to reflect more deeply upon the assumptions that you have brought into the situation. In particular, it will be necessary for your reflections to possess a critical element that enables you to uncover the knowledge, the values and the beliefs that you have assumed to be the case and that were influencing what you did, what you thought and what you felt about the experience. In doing so, you will have to employ the variety of critical thinking skills and attributes discussed in the previous chapter in order to examine your assumptions critically; in particular, this demands that you ask searching and challenging questions about those assumptions and evaluate whether there are good reasons for holding them and, if you conclude that there are not, to investigate and consider the possibility of adopting an alternative perspective.

Activity 2.5   *Evidence-based practice and research*

The alternative perspective that Philippa is discovering as she critically reflects upon her experience with Leon is that which is closely associated with the Hearing Voices Network, a perspective influenced by the work of Marius Romme and Sandra Escher (1993, 2000). For this activity, explore the website of the Hearing Voices Network (**www.hearing-voices.org**).

- What are the aims of the Hearing Voices Network and, broadly speaking, how do they go about attempting to achieve those aims?

An outline answer is provided at the end of the chapter.

In critically reflecting upon her clinical experience with Leon, Philippa is not simply identifying the assumptions that are influencing what she thinks, feels and does in that situation, but she is also questioning and evaluating the legitimacy and the value of those assumptions. While she thinks that some of her assumptions are appropriate, she is discovering that there are alternative perspectives which maintain differing assumptions and she is contemplating whether adopting these may be more effective in understanding and responding to Leon's experience of hearing voices. It is important to recognise that identifying, questioning and potentially changing your knowledge, values and beliefs as a result of critical reflection upon your clinical experiences – to engage in what has been referred to as a *perspective transformation* (Mezirow 1991) – can be both personally and professionally challenging. As highlighted in the previous chapter, you should not underestimate how attached you can become to your existing ways of understanding and doing things and critical reflection will therefore not only require you to use the intellectual skills, but also the range of emotional attributes that are associated with critical thinking. In particular, critical reflection requires you to become curious and inquisitive about your practice and the assumptions that underlie that practice, as well as maintaining the courage to question, challenge and change those assumptions if they do not withstand critical examination. Doing so will not only require you to become increasingly aware of your own knowledge, values and beliefs, but also to display humility in recognising the current limits of your understanding and a receptiveness to new ideas and perspectives. While it may be difficult to acknowledge the current limitations of your knowledge and competence, or that it has been superseded by new knowledge, research or evidence, the NMC's (2015) Code is clear about the importance of recognising and working within the current limits of your competence. In order to provide a high standard of mental health nursing care, it is essential for you to recognise and acknowledge the limits of your current understanding, knowledge and skills and to engage in activities, such as critical reflection, that will help you develop your practice and improve the experiences of those who use mental health services.

Activity 2.6   *Reflection*

Having selected and given a detailed, balanced description of a clinical experience, attempt to reflect upon that experience critically by asking yourself, and responding to, a series of critical questions. In developing Borton's (1970) reflective framework, Rolfe (2011) has proposed the following cue questions that might help you:

- So what does this experience tell me about my attitudes, assumptions and beliefs?
- So what was going through my mind as I acted?
- So what did I base my actions on?
- So what other knowledge can I bring to the situation?
- So what could I have done to make it better?
- So what is my new understanding of the situation?
- So what broader issues arise from the situation?

As this activity is based on your own reflections, there is no outline answer at the end of the chapter.

Action

Case study

After further reflection upon her experience with Leon, Philippa is increasingly questioning her own assumptions about the voice-hearing experience and the interventions that she has been providing. Rather than being an indication of his deteriorating mental health, she is now wondering if Leon's 'preoccupation' with his voices may be an indication that he is striving to make sense of them and discover a frame of reference within which to understand those voices. She has investigated this alternative perspective on auditory hallucinations in more detail and believes there may be value in presenting information about it to Leon when they next meet; indeed, before discussing a review of his medication with the medical team, she feels that this change of approach may be more productive at this stage. She is a little apprehensive about adopting this new perspective and implementing its associated strategies because she is only just becoming more familiar with it. However, after discussing with a senior colleague how she might practically go about doing this, she believes that she has the necessary interpersonal skills to help Leon explore and develop a framework within which to understand his experience of hearing voices if he feels this may be worthwhile. This perspective also emphasises the importance of encouraging those who hear voices to meet other people with similar voice-hearing experiences in order to normalise the experience, reduce isolation and provide an opportunity to learn from one another. Philippa has discovered that there is a 'hearing voices group' not far from where Leon lives and she has also decided to provide him with information about this group and discuss whether he would be keen to attend.

While both a balanced description and a reflection that adopts a critical perspective on a clinical experience are necessary for the process of critical reflection, those two stages are not by themselves sufficient. Rather, the third stage of a critically reflective ERA cycle requires you to consider what action you will take as a consequence of your description and reflection on that experience. As Thompson and Thompson (2008, p. 27) make clear, *reflective activities need to be directly part and parcel of the practice world and not an activity limited to educational programmes one or more steps removed from the day-to-day activities of practice.* In particular, the action stage of critical reflection requires you to consider what actions you will take as a result of your reflective activity and how that will affect your mental health practice and the way in which you conduct yourself in the clinical area. Such action need not produce a transformation that is as potentially dramatic as that undergone by Philippa in the above case study, a transformation which leads you to consider adopting a new theoretical and practical perspective on an aspect of mental distress. Rather, it may be that, as a consequence of critically reflecting upon a clinical experience, there is a subtle shift in one or more of your assumptions about any aspect of contemporary mental health care, a change in what you thought or believed to be the case. However, it will be necessary to express how that change relates back to your mental health nursing practice and, ultimately, how that change has contributed to improving the experiences of those who use mental health services.

Activity 2.7   *Reflection*

Having identified an experience, described it in a balanced way and subjected it to critical reflection, now consider what action you will take as a consequence of your reflective activity. In developing Borton's (1970) reflective framework, Rolfe (2011) has proposed the following action-directed questions that might help you to devise and implement a possible plan of action:

- Now what do I need to do to improve the care of those who use mental health services?
- Now what broader issues need to be considered if this action is to be successful?
- Now what might be the consequences of this action?

As this activity is based on your own reflections, there is no outline answer at the end of the chapter.

Once you have devised and implemented your plan of action you will then have a new clinical experience upon which to reflect critically. This will provide you with the opportunity to evaluate the success of your actions by once again progressing through the three stages of experience, reflection and action. In particular, it will provide you with the opportunity to consider disseminating the process and the results of your critical reflection to your peers if the interventions that arose as a consequence of that reflection were seemingly successful; alternatively, your new clinical experience will enable you to reconsider what else might need to change, and what other steps you may need to take, if your interventions did not produce the results that you had envisioned.

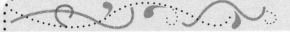

Chapter summary

In this chapter we have discussed the importance of critical reflection and why it is particularly important for you as you enter the rapidly changing and often disputed field of contemporary mental health care. Critical reflection has been distinguished from reflection by suggesting that the former requires you to adopt a critical perspective towards your clinical mental health practice experiences by employing the range of intellectual skills and emotional attributes associated with critical thinking. In particular, critical reflection has been presented as an activity in which your clinical experiences are considered in order to identify the assumptions that are influencing your thoughts, feelings and actions in those situations, and these are then rigorously questioned and challenged with a view to developing alternative ways of thinking, feeling and acting in future situations. While a variety of models and frameworks have been devised in order to help you engage in the process of critical reflection, this chapter has suggested that reflecting critically requires you to move through the three key stages of experience, reflection and action. In particular, it has encouraged you to begin employing these stages in order to reflect critically upon the range of clinical experiences that you have had, and that you will have, as a mental health nursing student and throughout your subsequent career as a mental health nurse; in doing so, you should now be in a position to begin to consider what your capabilities are with respect to critical reflection and how you can begin to develop as a critically reflective practitioner in contemporary mental health nursing.

Activities: brief outline answers

Activity 2.2 Critical thinking

Caitlin and William are expressing a number of commonly held and highly questionable assumptions about suicide and self-harm behaviours. These include the belief that people who talk about suicide and self-harm are not serious and will not engage in those behaviours, that talking to someone about those behaviours may inadvertently encourage that person to participate in them and that if a person is serious about suicide and self-harm then there is very little that can be done to prevent it (Santa Mina & Gallop 2009). Maintaining and perpetuating such assumptions could have disastrous consequences if they are not only influencing how Caitlin and William understand suicide and self-harm but also influencing their clinical interventions with those who use mental health services. In particular, those assumptions could be impairing Caitlin and William's mental health practice in a variety of ways; for example, it could be limiting their ability to assess suicide and self-harm risk competently, it could be inhibiting their ability to explore potential precipitating factors sufficiently and it could also be preventing them from exploring and promoting alternative coping strategies for those who are experiencing suicidal or self-harm ideation. It is important to remember that many people who have committed suicide or engaged in self-harm behaviours have spoken to someone beforehand and you should therefore always take such occurrences seriously; while such discussions can be both personally and professionally challenging, talking to a person about suicide and self-harm is one of the most important and potentially therapeutic interventions that you can provide as a mental health professional (Reeves 2010; Cutcliffe & Santos 2012; Roberts & Lamont 2014). Rather than encouraging participation in such behaviour, talking to a person about suicide and self-harm can give that person the permission to disclose thoughts and feelings of self-harm and suicide and this can ultimately enable a person to begin exploring alternative ways of coping with those thoughts and feelings.

Activity 2.5 Evidence-based practice and research

The aims of the Hearing Voices Network are:

- to raise awareness and acceptance of voice hearing, visions and other sensory experiences;

- to provide men, women and children who have these experiences with an opportunity to talk freely about this together;

- to support anyone with these experiences in seeking to understand, learn and grow from them in their own way.

In attempting to achieve these aims, the Hearing Voices Network employs a variety of strategies, such as promoting, developing and supporting Hearing Voices self-help groups; organising and delivering training sessions for health care workers and the general public; providing a forum to give men, women and children the opportunity to discuss voice hearing, visions and other sensory experiences; providing a confidential helpline that gives information and support to people with these experiences; and producing a newsletter that provides information on research, publications, personal accounts, coping strategies and creative pieces from those who hear voices.

Further reading

Howaston-Jones L (2013) *Reflective Practice in Nursing*, 2nd edition. London: Sage/Learning Matters.

An accessible introduction to reflective practice, this book provides numerous activities to help you develop the skills of reflection in the context of contemporary nursing practice.

Jasper M (2003) *Foundations in Nursing and Health Care: Beginning reflective practice*. Cheltenham: Nelson Thornes.

An established account of reflective practice in nursing and health care, this book introduces the ERA cycle and details the stages of experience, reflection and action as the essential components of reflection.

Rolfe G, Jasper M & Freshwater D (2011) *Critical Reflection in Practice*, 2nd edition. Basingstoke: Palgrave Macmillan.

This is a comprehensive and thought-provoking book on critical reflection that provides, among other things, a discussion of Schön's commonly overlooked notion of reflection-in-action.

Taylor BJ (2010) *Reflective Practice for Healthcare Professionals*, 3rd edition. Maidenhead: Open University Press.

This is a stimulating book that discusses three main types of reflection – technical reflection, practical reflection and emancipatory reflection – and draws on the work of the contemporary German philosopher Jürgen Habermas to inform that discussion.

Useful websites

www.flyingstart.scot.nhs.uk/learning-programmes/reflective-practice

This is the website for the Flying Start NHS programme, where you will find a variety of resources on reflective practice, including frameworks for reflection and practical strategies for engaging in reflective practice.

Chapter 3
Developing critical mental health practice

NMC Standards for Pre-registration Nursing Education

This chapter will address the following competencies:

Domain 3: Nursing practice and decision-making

10 All nurses must evaluate their care to improve clinical decision-making, quality and outcomes, using a range of methods, amending the plan of care, where necessary, and communicating changes to others.

Domain 4: Leadership, management and team working

1   All nurses must act as change agents and provide leadership through quality improvement and service development to enhance people's wellbeing and experiences of healthcare.

3   All nurses must be able to identify priorities and manage time and resources effectively to ensure the quality of care is maintained or enhanced.

6   All nurses must work independently as well as in teams. They must be able to take the lead in coordinating, delegating and supervising care safely, managing risk and remaining accountable for the care given.

7   All nurses must work effectively across professional and agency boundaries, actively involving and respecting others' contributions to integrated person-centred care. They must know when and how to communicate with and refer to other professionals and agencies in order to respect the choices of service users and others, promoting shared decision-making, to deliver positive outcomes and to coordinate smooth, effective transition within and between services and agencies.

Chapter aims

By the end of this chapter you will be able to:

- understand the importance of developing critical mental health practice;
- identify personal, social and institutional challenges to developing critical mental health practice;
- identify a range of constructive strategies for responding to those personal, social and institutional challenges.

Introduction

Case study

Nadia is midway through her mental health nursing programme and, so far, is really enjoying the course. Although she has found some of the lectures and tutorials challenging at times, she has particularly enjoyed those in which she has been given the opportunity to think critically about, and reflect critically upon, various aspects of contemporary mental health care. However, she is beginning to notice that on her clinical placements there doesn't appear to be many opportunities to consider critically how things could be done differently to improve the experiences of those who use mental health services. She has some ideas why this may be, but is unsure what she can do about it.

In the previous two chapters the activities of critical thinking and critical reflection have been examined. Both are essential for your academic studies as a mental health nursing student and throughout your subsequent career as a mental health nurse. The employment of the intellectual skills, emotional attributes and personal qualities that are associated with critical thinking and critical reflection will enable you to adopt a critical perspective towards contemporary mental health care. In particular, they will enable you, where necessary, to question, challenge and potentially change practice that does not withstand critical examination in order to ensure that your care is informed, accountable and responsive to the needs of those who use mental health services. However, like Nadia in the case study above, you may believe that critical thinking and critical reflection are sometimes limited in the clinical area, and you may even have identified potential barriers to engaging in such activity at the individual, group or even organisational level. Indeed, a number of obstacles to critical thinking and reflection have been identified in the literature, including anxiety about, and a lack of confidence in, one's critical abilities; an under-appreciation of the value of critical thinking and reflection, and particularly its value for 'everyday' practice; a reluctance and apprehension to question existing practices and those individuals perceived as experts or authorities, and it has even been suggested that there exists an implicit, or sometimes explicit, hostility to critical thinking and critically reflective activities (Thompson & Thompson 2008; Taylor 2010; Cottrell 2011). While such challenges may sometimes be a source of frustration and disappointment, they should not be a source of despair. Many mental health nurses are continually seeking to develop, refine and incorporate critical thinking and critical reflection into their everyday work and, by doing so, engage in what we will refer to throughout this chapter as critical mental health practice. As a mental health nursing student in an academic setting that is receptive to, and stresses the importance of, critical thinking and reflection, you have a unique opportunity to begin to incorporate those activities into your work and, by doing so, begin to consider how you can develop your own critical mental health practice.

The purpose of this chapter is to introduce you to the notion of critical mental health practice and to enable you to consider how you can begin to develop such practice. In particular, it will discuss how your engagement in critical thinking and critical reflection may be limited, to a greater or lesser extent, by a variety of personal, social and institutional obstacles. While you may encounter multiple and diverse challenges to such critical activity, this chapter will examine four that can be understood as being representative of the variety of obstacles that can potentially limit the incorporation of critical thinking and reflection into your mental health practice. First, it will discuss common and enduring misunderstandings about the character and purpose of critical thinking and reflection; second, it will examine what is referred to as **egocentrism**, the tendency to perceive things exclusively from our own perspective and in accordance with our own interests; third, it will consider how the organisations within which mental health nurses work can obstruct participation in critical mental health practice; and finally, it will discuss how resources can limit the opportunities to integrate critical thinking and reflection into that practice. By doing so, this chapter will encourage you to review your own situation and to consider the limitations, restrictions and challenges that may confront you in your own particular case. While there are rarely simple solutions to these often diverse and complex challenges, you will also be encouraged to think about adopting and developing constructive strategies to address such challenges and, ultimately, how this can enable you to incorporate critical thinking and critical reflection into your mental health practice.

Misunderstandings

One of the most significant challenges that you may encounter as you seek to incorporate critical thinking and reflection into your mental health practice will concern common misunderstandings surrounding the character and the purpose of those activities. These misunderstandings may be diverse and can often occur at the individual level, but they can also be misunderstandings held by groups of people, such as nursing teams, and they can even be present throughout the culture of a whole organisation. Such misunderstandings may involve, for example, a lack of knowledge about what intellectual skills and emotional attributes are required to engage in critical thinking and reflection or the degree to which they require an examination, and potential transformation, of the assumptions underlying our thoughts, feelings and actions. However, arguably the most widespread and enduring misunderstanding about critical thinking and critical reflection, and which is therefore a particularly challenging misunderstanding to address, involves the perception of those activities as being concerned with criticism and criticising. In particular, such critical activity is often characterised as a negative and even destructive endeavour whose purpose is to criticise and find fault with the thoughts, feelings and actions of others without offering anything constructive in return. Those who participate in such activities can be presented in a negative, stereotypical way as being mischievous or even resentful people who seek to cause annoyance and disruption, or as people who see themselves as superior and seek to ridicule the supposedly naïve, misguided and even mistaken opinions and practices of others. Indeed, it has been suggested that *Being critical is seen to have harmful consequences, such as destroying others' motivation or causing irreparable harm to their self-image* (Brookfield 2001, p. 35). Therefore, one of the most significant challenges that you will encounter as you attempt to incorporate critical thinking and critical reflection into your mental health practice will be to address the misunderstanding of those activities as being concerned with criticising and, as a consequence, as activities that are to be treated with suspicion or even outright hostility.

Case study

Kofi is in the fifth week of his clinical placement on an older adult mental health ward. His mentor has a keen interest in critical reflection and she has been encouraging Kofi to reflect on, and seek to develop, his communication skills when interacting with those people with dementia. In order to facilitate this, she has appointed herself as Kofi's 'critical friend'. However, as part of this process of critical reflection he can recall being told on various occasions that his communication skills are 'a little rudimentary' and that he is not at the level where he should be. While he has asked how he might begin to develop his ability to communicate with those with dementia he cannot recall being given much support or instruction apart from being told to 'pay more attention' to the qualified staff. This is the first time that he has encountered the notion and the practice of critical reflection and, needless to say, he is finding it to be a largely unproductive and negative experience.

In considering Kofi's experience in the above case study, you may suspect that his mentor has misunderstood critical reflection to be an activity that involves criticising others and, as a consequence, that this is leading Kofi to begin to associate such critical activity with criticism. While critical reflection and critical thinking, along with many other practices and procedures in contemporary mental health care, can be used as pretence to engage in the criticism of others, it is important to note that there is no necessary connection between those critical activities and engaging in criticism. As you seek to incorporate such critical activity into your mental health practice, it will be necessary to develop and maintain a clear distinction between the two in your own mind and in your own practice; to maintain a clear distinction between those critical activities that seek to facilitate insights and positive change and any other activities that lead others, either intentionally or unintentionally, to feel that they are being criticised, disregarded or disparaged. As we have discussed over the previous two chapters, a central characteristic of critical thinking and reflection is the ability to ask challenging questions, both of oneself and of others, in order to examine the validity and appropriateness of existing assumptions and practices in contemporary mental health care. In doing so, however, it is important to recognise that many people may feel uncomfortable, anxious or even threatened by such critical activity and it will be necessary, as far as is possible, to take steps to minimise such effects. Indeed, it has been suggested that the challenge facing anyone who would engage in critical thinking and critical reflection is to consider how to communicate the character, purpose and results of those activities *in ways which build relationships rather than damaging them; which expand consciousness rather than causing it to constrict under the influence of shame, fear or humiliation* (Heath 2012, p. 14).

Activity 3.1   *Decision making*

Consider Kofi's experience in the case study above and the manner in which his mentor appears to have understood the character and purpose of being a critical friend. The role of a critical friend to facilitate critical thinking and reflection has been identified as a valuable one insofar as critical friends can ask important questions and provide alternative perspectives that can lead to fresh insights and more sophisticated reflections (Taylor 2010).

continued ...

In contrast to Kofi's mentor, decide how you would have performed the role of being his critical friend in order to encourage him to reflect upon and develop his communication skills with those with dementia. In particular, what would you have avoided doing as his critical friend and what alternative values, qualities and styles of communicating would you have employed?

An outline answer is provided at the end of the chapter.

Egocentrism

Another considerable challenge that you may encounter as you seek to incorporate critical thinking and critical reflection into your mental health practice will be egocentrism. The notion of egocentrism has been employed in a variety of areas and disciplines and it is an important notion in, for example, Jean Piaget's (1959) account of childhood cognitive development; in particular, it is employed to characterise how young children, in the preoperational stage of development, are understood as being unable to distinguish their perspective from the perspective of others. In the context of critical thinking and reflection, however, egocentrism has a broader application and refers to the tendency of any person, irrespective of age, to think, feel and act exclusively from his or her own perspective without giving due consideration to alternative perspectives (Paul & Elder 2014). While it can be a characteristic trait of any individual, it can also manifest itself at the collective level such that a group of people can adhere to a particular perspective in which the potential limitations of that perspective, and the potential strengths of other perspectives, are overlooked or actively disregarded.

Case study

Catherine is a third-year mental health nursing student on clinical placement within a community mental health team. She has found that many members of the team favour an understanding and response to mental distress by employing a cognitive behavioural approach. Her mentor has told her that the team leader is a 'vigorous supporter' of this approach and almost all of the staff have attended some form of training course in cognitive behavioural therapy. Catherine is keen to deepen her understanding of this approach but has informed her mentor that, as part of completing her practice assessment document, she is also required to display an understanding of a variety of approaches to understanding and responding to mental distress. Her mentor has suggested that they can discuss these but they are now 'largely irrelevant' in contemporary mental health care and, in thinking about her personal and professional development, she ought to concentrate on developing her knowledge and skills surrounding cognitive behavioural therapy.

Egocentrism, the tendency to adhere to a single perspective without giving due consideration to alternative perspectives, presents a significant obstacle to the development of critical mental health practice. The ability to reflect critically upon your own perspective – to think critically about your current understanding and approach to mental distress, and consider alternative ways of understanding and doing things – is essential to becoming an informed, proactive professional who is responsive to the diverse needs of those who use mental health services. However, there may be multiple reasons why a person or even a group of people may adhere to a single perspective without giving due consideration to others. It will therefore be important for you to ask critical questions of yourself periodically to prevent your practice becoming limited by, and even 'entrenched' within, a single perspective. For example, do you adhere to your own perspective because you fear that considering alternative perspectives may expose your own as inconsistent, inappropriate or even ineffective? Do you disregard other perspectives on mental health and distress because the one that you hold is shared by others and, in particular, by people in positions of authority or by people that you respect professionally? Or do you engage in possible egocentric ways of thinking and behaving because it is in your own self-interest to do so and it provides you with, for example, some form of personal or professional advantage? In order to develop your own critical mental health practice it will not only be necessary for you to gain an awareness of the potential reasons for why you may engage in egocentrism, but it will also be necessary to maintain a curiosity about, and receptiveness towards, alternative perspectives and approaches to mental health care. In particular, it will require you to gain an appreciation of the complexity of mental health and distress and to develop an awareness that adopting different perspectives, and employing a plurality of therapeutic approaches, will enable you to respond to the distress of different people at different times (Cooper & McLeod 2011). As we discussed in Chapter 1, this does not mean that you are ready to accept any perspective or that all perspectives are equally valid, but it does mean that you are receptive to new ideas and approaches from a variety of sources and you are willing to subject those alternative ideas and approaches to critical consideration.

Activity 3.2   *Reflection*

A productive way to prevent your mental health practice becoming limited by, and even entrenched within, a single perspective is actively to explore alternative perspectives. You may already be aware that there are a number of theoretical frameworks or conceptual models that seek to account for how mental distress arises and what are therefore the most appropriate means to respond to that distress. Established models include, for example, the biological or what is often referred to as the medical model, the humanistic or existential model, the psychodynamic model, the cognitive model, the behavioural model and the social model. However, it is not unusual to develop a preference for one perspective over the others and you may already have done so without giving due consideration to the strengths of other perspectives, or the limitations of the model that you favour.

For this activity, determine which model you have a preference for and choose an alternative model upon which to reflect. As you do so, maintain a curiosity about, and receptiveness towards, that alternative perspective by identifying its potential strengths and how it may help you to respond to the diverse needs of those who use mental health services.

As this activity is based on your own reflections, there is no outline answer at the end of the chapter.

Organisations

A significant proportion, if not all, of the care that you provide during your time as a mental health nursing student, and subsequently throughout your career as a qualified mental health nurse, will occur within the context of health care organisations. While doing so will almost certainly have beneficial consequences for your personal and professional development, it is important to recognise that organisational settings may also present a number of limitations to developing and maintaining critical mental health practice. While diverse challenges may exist, many are likely to be a manifestation of a conflict between the concerns, objectives or culture of the organisation in which you will work and your attempt to promote and incorporate critical thinking and critical reflection into your practice. While understanding an entity as complex as an organisation can be particularly problematic, it has been suggested that many modern health care organisations are increasingly characterised by what has been referred to as **managerialism** and, in particular, by the ongoing drive to maximise efficiency in order to achieve certain targets (Thompson & Thompson 2008). In the context of such an approach, mental health professionals can come to be characterised as being employed to carry out their employer's instructions: as being required to follow the instructions of the organisation's managers rather than as professional practitioners with the knowledge, skills and experience to resolve problems and make decisions with a significant degree of autonomy. In a climate focused on 'getting things done', on maximising efficiency and achieving targets, critical thinking and reflection can come to be regarded as an unaffordable luxury at best and, at worst, as a dangerous challenge to the aims, objectives and efficient functioning of the organisation. Indeed, while the critical examination of existing ways of doing and understanding things can lead to positive change and development for both individuals and the organisation within which they work, Schön (1983, p. 328) has suggested that such a critically reflective practitioner can also become, *by the same token, a danger to the stable system of rules and procedures within which [s]he is expected to deliver [her]his technical expertise.*

Concept summary: Images of organisation

Attempting to understand an entity as complex as a health care organisation can be a considerable challenge. In order to do so, however, a number of similes, metaphors or images are commonly used and these can influence how you understand the impact of the organisation within which you work on your practice and what you believe is possible within that organisation. For example, in *Images of Organization*, Gareth Morgan (2006) identifies a number of common images that are used to understand organisations, including:

- organisations as machines that are designed to achieve particular objectives in an efficient, reliable and predictable way. The tasks required to achieve those objectives are clearly determined and the members of the organisation, understood as parts of the machine, are expected to carry them out in a largely uncritical and unreflective manner;

(Continued)

(Continued)

- organisations as organisms that are understood as living systems and are required to change, adapt and evolve in order to survive. The members of that organisation, analogous to the cells of an organism, are valued insofar as they are essential to the growth, innovation and evolution of the organisation as a whole;
- organisations as political systems that seek to govern their members according to a range of political strategies and principles (e.g. by **democratic**, **autocratic** or **technocratic** means). In particular, organisations as political systems seek to manage the individual and collective interests or agendas of their members and to address the complex issues of power, conflict and authority.
- organisations as psychic prisons that develop favoured ways of thinking and doing things. While these can be productive, the members of the organisation can become caught, entrenched or even 'imprisoned' within these favoured ways of thinking and doing things and, therefore, unwilling to consider alternative perspectives.

Responding to how an organisation's concerns, objectives or culture can limit the promotion and incorporation of critical thinking and reflection into mental health practice can be a significant challenge. To propose that there is a simple strategy that will enable you to do so is to underestimate the sometimes considerable complexity of attempting to facilitate change within an organisational context. Over the course of your mental health nursing programme you will learn about the theory and practice of managing change in health care organisations and this will help you think about how to develop your critical mental health practice. However, a number of 'everyday' strategies for responding to the organisational challenges surrounding the integration of critical thinking and reflection into workplace settings have been identified and you should consider how you can begin to incorporate these into your work (Brookfield 2001; Thompson & Thompson 2008; Taylor 2010). One of the most important and potentially influential of these strategies which is immediately available to you is the practice of **modelling**, **embodying** or **leading by example**. In particular, you can begin to affirm your worth as a critical mental health practitioner by discussing with others, and embodying in your practice, how critical thinking and critical reflection enable you to be a more informed and accountable practitioner who is responsive to the diverse needs of those who use mental health services. While you may encounter resistance as you do so, you should remember that in every organisation there will almost certainly be people who resist unreflective and routine practice and will do so in a variety of ways: in a quiet, subtle and unobtrusive manner or in more overt, public and assertive ways (Heath 2012). In embodying critical mental health practice you will attract the interest of others within your organisation who share, or who aspire to develop, a similar disposition. You should work towards ensuring that you make productive, mutually respectful alliances with these colleagues, irrespective of the professional body to which they belong, so that you are able to assist each other in facilitating the development of critical thinking and critical reflection in contemporary mental health care.

Activity 3.3 — *Critical thinking*

How you understand the organisation within which you provide mental health care will influence your assessment of the impact of that organisation on your practice and what you believe is possible within that setting. For this activity, critically consider the common similes, metaphors and images used to think about organisations that have been summarised above.

- Do you understand the organisation in which you practise in a similar way to one, or perhaps a combination, of these images?
- If not, how do you understand the organisation within which you provide mental health care?
- Based on your understanding of that organisation, what opportunities do you think exist for you to incorporate critical thinking and reflection into your practice and how might you go about doing so in that setting?

As this activity is based on your own critical thinking, there is no outline answer at the end of the chapter.

Resources

An enduring challenge to the incorporation of critical thinking and critical reflection into your mental health practice, and to the provision of quality mental health care more generally, concerns resources and a lack of resources in particular. Resources are often understood in tangible, material terms and, in health care settings, are commonly understood to refer to things such as money, equipment or the numbers of available staff. However, it is important to recognise that some of the most valuable resources available to you can exist in an intangible or non-material form and can include, for example, knowledge, motivation and time. Indeed, while you are now actively developing your knowledge about critical thinking and reflection, a potential obstacle to the incorporation of these activities into your practice will concern constraints on your time which, in turn, can lead to a loss of motivation to engage in such critical activities. Developing your time management skills and remaining motivated and committed to developing your mental health practice will be important aspects of your academic and clinical training as you progress through your course. Multiple practical strategies have been proposed to enable you to do so, including the identification and employment of critical friends, the creation of daily critical thinking and reflection routines and the development of supportive critical networks both within and beyond your immediate working environment (Taylor 2010; Howatson-Jones 2013). However, as you are probably already aware, the environments within which contemporary mental health care is provided can be busy, challenging and high-pressured and it is possible to develop a sense that you are being 'caught up and swept along' by the sometimes frenetic pace of those settings. When this occurs you can begin to feel overwhelmed by the demands that are being placed upon you and this, in turn, can lead you to feel that there is simply not the time to incorporate critical thinking and reflection into your busy mental health practice.

··

Case study

Dylan has been a mental health nurse for over 20 years and has encountered many ideas and initia-tives designed to improve mental health practice in that time. One of those whose value he can appre-ciate is critical thinking and reflection, but he maintains that there is never enough time to incorporate those activities seriously into his busy schedule as a community mental health nurse. Today, for exam-ple, he had put time aside in the morning to reflect on an incident earlier in the week with Janet, the second-year mental health nursing student. However, the morning team meeting over-ran by an hour and then he agreed to go on an unscheduled joint visit with another member of staff. He attempted to rearrange his meeting with Janet for later in the afternoon but, after driving into town to have lunch, completing the case notes that he should have done earlier in the week and then getting caught up in a discussion with the team leader for over an hour, there was no time left for anything else.

··

Almost certainly there will be occasions when busy working schedules may only permit the brief-est of opportunities to participate in critical thinking and critical reflection. On other occasions, however, it may be that the sense of being too busy to engage in those activities is a mistaken perception and not an accurate, balanced evaluation of the time that is available to you. This can potentially be the consequence of working within a culture that understands work as 'doing, not thinking' and that contributes to a collective, enduring and overwhelming sense that *there are never enough hours in the day* (Thompson & Thompson 2008). A productive intervention that will enable you progressively to achieve a degree of **non-attachment** from such a cultural and collec-tive sense and, in doing so, will assist you in making more accurate evaluations of the time that is available to engage in critical thinking and reflection is the use of mindfulness-based tech-niques. Indeed, there now exists an emerging body of literature that not only discusses mindful-ness as a psychotherapeutic intervention (Williams *et al.* 2007; Roberts 2015), but also as an intervention that can, among other things, enable you to acquire a clearer perspective on the obstacles and opportunities in your working environment (Arpa 2013). In addition, a particu-larly useful intervention that can help you to make more accurate evaluations of the time availa-ble to you in your working schedule, and which can complement mindfulness-based techniques, is what is referred to as the CIA model, where CIA is an initialism for control, influence and accept (Thompson & Thompson 2008). In the context of attempting to determine where there may be opportunities in your schedule to engage in critical thinking and reflection, the CIA model requires you to make a clear assessment of what you can control, what you can influence and what, being unable currently to control or influence, you may have to accept.

Activity 3.4   *Team working*

··

The CIA model can be a particularly helpful tool in assisting you to organise your working schedule in busy environments and to maximise the opportunities for participating in critical thinking and critical reflection. In particular, it can highlight what is directly within your control to change and it can encourage you to generate strategic and creative ways to

continued . . .

influence your working environment so that you can develop and maintain critical mental health practice. In addition, it can help you to accept what you are currently unable to control or influence and to focus your energies in productive ways on what is within your sphere of control and influence.

Consider the case study above and, with your colleagues, apply the CIA model to Dylan's working day. In doing so, attempt to determine where he might have been able to create an opportunity to engage in a 30-minute period of critical thinking and reflection by identifying what he could have controlled, what he might have been able to influence and what he may have had to accept.

An outline answer is provided at the end of the chapter.

Chapter summary

This chapter has identified the importance of critical mental health practice and has considered how you can begin to develop such practice. It has suggested that you may encounter a variety of limitations, restrictions and challenges when seeking to incorporate critical thinking and critical reflection into your mental health practice and these may manifest at a personal, social and even institutional level. In particular, four significant challenges have been identified which can be understood as being representative of the many, diverse challenges that you may confront. First, it has discussed the common and enduring misunderstanding that critical thinking and reflection are characterised by criticism and criticising; second, it has examined that which is referred to as egocentrism, the tendency to perceive things exclusively from our own perspective and in accordance with our own interests; third, it has considered the potential conflict between critical mental health practice and the concerns, objectives or culture of the organisation in which mental health care is provided; and finally, it has discussed how resources, and time constraints in particular, may limit the opportunities to engage in critical thinking and reflection. In doing so, this chapter has sought to encourage you to review your own situation and to consider the limitations, restrictions and challenges that may confront you in your own particular case. While there are rarely simple solutions to these often diverse and complex challenges, this chapter has discussed, and encouraged you to begin to consider adopting and developing, a number of constructive strategies to respond to the challenge of incorporating critical thinking and critical reflection into your mental health practice.

Activities: brief outline answers

Activity 3.1 Decision making

In deciding how you would have performed the role of being Kofi's critical friend, you may have stressed the importance of not criticising him or behaving in ways that could be understood as criticism. The role of being a critical friend places as much emphasis on the 'friend' aspect of the role as it does on its 'critical' aspect and, in doing so, aims to encourage others to think critically about their practice in supportive, non-threatening and enabling ways. To do this, you may have identified that it is important to work towards building relationships with others in which there is a sense of respect and trust; rather than being directive and telling people what you think is wrong with their practice and what they should do about it, you may have identified that it is more productive to create a climate in which people are allowed to talk freely about, and are encouraged to make sense of, their own clinical experiences and potential areas of development. To facilitate this process you may have suggested a variety of communication skills such as the use of **paraphrasing**, reflecting and summarising what others say, along with the employment of appropriately timed, **open questions** and supportive comments to encourage deeper levels of critical thinking and reflection. Finally, while recognising that such critical activity can involve making evaluations and tentative suggestions about the merits of the various assumptions, beliefs and practices maintained by others, you may also have noted the importance of striving to remain non-judgemental about the other as a person.

Activity 3.4 Team working

In applying the CIA model to Dylan's working day and considering where he could have created an opportunity to engage in critical thinking and reflection, you may have identified that there are no simple answers about what he could have controlled, what he might have been able to influence and what he may have had to accept. For example, you may have had interesting discussions with your colleagues surrounding the possibility of Dylan being able to control, influence or accept the manner in which the morning team meeting over-ran by an hour. Could he have controlled the situation by excusing himself and leaving the meeting at the time it was originally intended to finish? Could he have influenced the situation, and the possibility of the team meeting over-running in the future, by attempting to gain an agreement that it ought to finish at the intended time and that, for example, any non-urgent business is to be carried over to the next team meeting? Or was it that things had to be discussed in this morning's team meeting that required more time and, on this occasion, it was something that Dylan simply had to accept? Similarly, you may have had interesting discussions about the application of the CIA model to a number of incidents that occurred throughout Dylan's working day, including the unscheduled joint visit with a colleague, his drive into town for lunch, the completion of the case notes and the lengthy discussion that he had in the afternoon with the team leader.

Further reading

Cooper M & McLeod J (2011) *Pluralistic Counselling and Psychotherapy*. London: Sage.

This is a stimulating and accessible book that stresses the importance, and celebrates the value, of adopting different perspectives and pluralistic approaches to counselling and psychotherapy.

Hewitt-Taylor J (2013) *Understanding and Managing Change in Healthcare: A step-by-step guide*. Basingstoke: Palgrave Macmillan.

A comprehensive account of how to plan, implement, maintain and evaluate change in modern health care settings, as well as an informative discussion about barriers to change and how they might be overcome.

Paul R & Elder L (2014) *Critical Thinking: Tools for taking charge of your professional and personal life*, 2nd edition. Upper Saddle River, NJ: Pearson Education.

This is a comprehensive and detailed work that discusses many aspects of critical thinking and which provides, among other things, an informative discussion about understanding, monitoring and tackling egocentrism.

Thompson S & Thompson N (2008) *The Critically Reflective Practitioner*. Basingstoke: Palgrave Macmillan.

A succinct and engaging book on the theoretical and practical aspects of critical reflection that includes a discussion about the variety of obstacles facing the incorporation of critical reflection into health and social care practice.

Useful websites

www.bemindful.co.uk

This is the website for the Mental Health Foundation that provides information on mindfulness-based cognitive therapy and mindfulness-based stress reduction, and that also provides a variety of mindfulness-based resources and online exercises.

www.nhs.uk/Conditions/stress-anxiety-depression/Pages/Time-management-tips.aspx

Here you will find the website for NHS Choices that provides a number of accessible time management strategies that can be incorporated into your daily mental health nursing practice.

Chapter 4
Self and values

Chapter aims

By the end of this chapter you will be able to:

- define values and **values-based practice** in mental health nursing;
- identify the importance of recognising, and working with, your personal values, the professional values of mental health nursing and the values of those who use mental health services;
- understand contemporary critical discussions about the presence of values in the identification of mental distress;
- identify the significance and implication of these critical discussions for contemporary mental health nursing practice.

Introduction

Case study

Maylin is a second-year mental health nursing student who is currently speaking to her tutor about an essay that she is writing on working in a collaborative, person-centred way with those who use mental health services. Maylin's tutor has suggested that she may want to include a critical discussion about values into her work and he has advised her not only to identify the importance of recognising values in mental health nursing but also the challenges that practitioners may face when working with values. In particular, he has stressed the need to discuss how working with values in contemporary mental health care requires practitioners to identify and work with their own personal values, the professional values of mental health nursing and the values of those who use mental health services. Maylin has taken note of her tutor's suggestions but, reflecting on the meeting as she walks home, begins to recognise that she has only the vaguest notion of what values are.

As a mental health nursing student you will have undoubtedly been introduced to the importance of developing therapeutic relationships and supportive alliances with those who use mental health services. One of the most important elements in the establishment of such relationships, and your mental health practice more generally, will therefore be you – who you are as an individual person and practitioner – or what is more precisely referred to as your 'self'. In order to develop your ability to establish therapeutic relationships through the employment of who you are – what is commonly referred to as 'the therapeutic use of self' – you will have begun to learn about and practise a whole range of verbal and non-verbal communication skills. However, in order to deepen your ability to establish supportive relationships through the therapeutic use of self, and not only to appreciate what facilitates but also what can restrict this process, it will be necessary for you to begin to think critically about and reflect upon your beliefs, your attitudes and, importantly, your values. Indeed, there is a growing awareness in contemporary mental health nursing of the importance of values and, in particular, of the manner in which they can profoundly influence, in both productive and non-productive ways, how we think about and respond to the experiences of those who use mental health services (McLean *et al.* 2012; Stacey & Diamond 2014). In order to become a self-aware mental health practitioner who is able to establish supportive, therapeutic relationships with others, it will therefore be necessary for you to consider both the impact of your personal values, and the values of mental health nursing more generally, upon your practice. However, in order to become a mental health practitioner who is responsive to the needs of people who experience mental distress, it will also be important for you to begin to gain an awareness of, and work collaboratively with, the values of those who use mental health services.

The purpose of this chapter is to introduce you to the notion of values and the significance of values in contemporary mental health care. In particular, it will begin by providing a provisional definition of values before encouraging you to reflect critically upon your personal values and to think critically about the professional values of mental health nursing. While consideration of personal and professional values is central to your ability to establish therapeutic relationships with others, we shall examine the importance of gaining an awareness of, and ability to begin to work with, the values of those who use mental health services, and we shall do so within the context of 'values-based practice' in mental health nursing. However, critical discussions about the presence of values in contemporary mental health care extend beyond the recognition of the importance of practising in a values-based manner. One of the most enduring and significant of these discussions is concerned with the role that values play in understanding and conceptualising the experiences of those who use mental health services. This chapter will therefore not only introduce you to the ideas and debates that characterise that discussion, but will also encourage you to begin to appreciate, reflect upon and critically engage with that discussion. Doing so will not only enable you to begin to develop deeper levels of critical thinking and critical reflection for your academic studies, but will also enable you to think more critically about the assumptions, attitudes and beliefs that inform your own mental health nursing practice.

Values

Although you may have encountered discussions about the importance of recognising and working with values in mental health nursing, you may, like Maylin in the case study above, be unsure what values are. If this is the case, then it might be reassuring to know that the nature of values has been widely discussed and disputed for many years and developing a clear understanding of what values are can be particularly challenging, not least because of the manner in which they are closely connected to a number of other notions, such as beliefs, **norms** and **ethics**. Despite these challenges, however, values can provisionally be understood as referring to that which we deem to be worthy, important or desirable and, in doing so, can often reveal what are our deepest goals, ambitions and priorities (Table 4.1). Indeed, in revealing what we consider to be worthy and desirable, it has been suggested that one of the most important characteristics of values is the manner in which they also influence our decisions and actions (Hare 1952; Fulford 2008). We can see this if we consider compassion, a value that has not only gained increased attention in the nursing literature but has also been central to current debates about health care policy, practice and education (DH 2012; Dewar *et al.* 2014; Stickley & Spandler 2014). If compassion is a value that we personally deem to be worthy and desirable, then we may also believe that it is important to be considerate and caring towards others. Holding compassion as an important value may not only influence our everyday decisions and conduct, but may also influence our longer-term goals and ambitions, including, for example, our decision to pursue a career in mental health nursing.

In seeking to deepen your understanding of what values are, it is important to recognise that they have been said to possess a number of varying characteristics (McLean *et al.* 2012; Stacey & Diamond 2014). For example, while values may influence our decisions and our actions in profound ways, we may have adopted them with minimal reflection and be only partially aware of their presence. However, it is possible to make our values explicit and, in doing so, reflect upon, revise or reject our existing values and adopt alternative ones from a variety of sources. In addition, while values can be

Accountability	Happiness	Power
Achievement	Honesty	Privacy
Adventure	Independence	Recognition
Autonomy	Individuality	Reliability
Collaboration	Initiative	Responsibility
Commitment	Integrity	Security
Compassion	Intelligence	Self-awareness
Competition	Intimacy	Sincerity
Creativity	Knowledge	Solitude
Decisiveness	Leadership	Spirituality
Determination	Learning	Stability
Discipline	Love	Status
Diversity	Loyalty	Strength
Efficiency	Modesty	Success
Equality	Money	Tolerance
Faith	Obedience	Trust
Family	Perfection	Truth
Flexibility	Persistence	Unity
Friendship	Pleasure	Wealth
Generosity	Positivity	Wisdom

Table 4.1: Common personal values

shared by individuals, they can also vary among people and it is possible for differing values to conflict, not only between people but also within a single individual. Finally, some of our values can be comparatively stable, values that we may hold over the course of our lifetime and that can express who and what we are in a fundamental way – what are sometimes referred to as 'core values'. In contrast, we can possess values that are less fundamental to our self-conceptions and identity – what are sometimes referred to as 'secondary' values – and which are more liable to change over the course of our lifetime and in response to changing circumstances.

Activity 4.1   *Reflection*

Both as a mental health nursing student, and throughout your career as a mental health nurse, it will be important for you to think critically about and reflect upon your personal values. As you are probably already aware, a fundamental feature of mental health nursing

continued . . .

is the ability to establish therapeutic relationships and supportive, enabling alliances with those who use mental health services. This will require you, among other things, to develop significant levels of self-awareness and an important aspect of this is the ability to recognise how your personal values may affect your ability to establish supportive relationships in both productive and less productive ways.

For this activity, consider the list of common personal values provided in Table 4.1. As you do so, identify three core values – three values that are very important to you, and two secondary values – values that are still important to you but perhaps not as important as the previous three (if you identify values that are not on the list, then you can use these instead). For each of your values, consider how they might affect your interactions with those who use mental health services in positive, productive ways and also consider if they may affect those interactions in a less positive and productive manner.

As this activity is based on your own reflections, there is no outline answer at the end of the chapter.

Mental health nursing and professional values

While reflecting upon and thinking critically about your personal values is an important aspect of developing your self-awareness, and therefore your mental health nursing practice, as you progress through your course you will be introduced, whether in an implicit or an explicit way, to the values of nursing as a profession. Partly as a consequence of a number of investigations into high-profile health care failings – such as that evidenced at the Mid-Staffordshire NHS Foundation Trust – there has been an increased emphasis on making the professional values of nursing explicit. For example, you may have been introduced to the Department of Health's (2012) *Compassion in Practice,* which explicitly identifies six fundamental values – the so-called '6Cs' of care, compassion, competence, communication, courage and commitment – that it suggests ought to underpin the work of all nurses. Similarly, the NMC's (2015) Code can also be understood as a statement of the fundamental values that ought to guide your work in so far as it asserts the value of prioritising people, practising effectively, preserving safety and promoting professionalism and trust. In addition to such explicit statements about the professional values of nursing generally, however, an important question for you to consider is whether there are professional values that are particular to mental health nursing. As we have already identified, it has been suggested that what is distinctive about mental health nursing is the value attached to developing and maintaining therapeutic relationships and, in order to achieve this, the value of developing empathy, displaying genuineness and demonstrating acceptance or unconditional positive regard (Rogers 1957, 2004). More recently, it has been suggested that the values of mental health nursing reside in the ability not only to provide physical and emotional security to people who are experiencing periods of acute distress, but also to foster an atmosphere of hope, optimism and the belief that recovery is possible (Barker 2009a; Barker & Buchanan-Barker 2009).

Activity 4.2	*Team working*

A number of policy documents have sought to identify explicitly the professional values of mental health nursing, and the values and capabilities of those who work in contemporary mental health care more generally (DH 2004, 2006; Scottish Executive 2006). These have included the need to:

- respect diversity;
- promote recovery;
- challenge inequality;
- work collaboratively;
- combat **stigma**;
- provide meaningful choices;
- promote social inclusion;
- practise ethically;
- enable positive risk taking.

Attempting to determine what professional values mean in practice, however, can be a particular challenge because they can be interpreted differently by different practitioners depending on the context or the variety of settings in which they work. With your colleagues choose one of the values listed above and attempt to gain a consensus on what it means in contemporary mental health practice. In particular, identify how adopting this value would influence, in practical ways, your work with those who use mental health services.

As this activity is based on your own reflections, there is no outline answer at the end of the chapter.

Values-based practice in mental health nursing

Critically thinking about and reflecting upon the professional values of mental health nursing, and attempting to determine what those values might mean in practice, will enable you to develop an increasing understanding of the overarching purpose, aims and objectives of your chosen field of health care. However, in order to become a mental health practitioner who is responsive to the needs of those who use mental health services, it will be important for you also to begin to recognise and work with the values of others. Indeed, in recent years the notion of values-based practice has been introduced into mental health nursing, in which there is an explicit acknowledgement that our own personal values, our professional values and the values of those who use mental health services are all inextricably involved in every aspect of our clinical practice and decision making (Fulford *et al.* 2012; McLean *et al.* 2012).

Values-based practice is a complex, multidimensional notion that provides a conceptual framework for thinking about the values that are present in contemporary mental health practice and also discusses the skills, qualities and attitudes that are important when working with the diversity of values that are present in any clinical situation (Fulford 2007). However, a productive way to begin to appreciate the importance of values-based practice in mental health nursing is to contrast it with evidence-based practice. As you progress through your mental health nursing programme you will almost certainly be introduced to the notion of evidence-based practice and you will gain an awareness that it involves the explicit use of the best current evidence when making decisions about which interventions and treatments to employ with those who use health care services (Sackett *et al.* 1996). However, exponents of values-based practice have suggested that, while evidence can indicate, with varying degrees of certainty, what will be the outcome of employing certain interventions and treatments, it does not enable us to determine if those outcomes will be valued from the individual perspective of any one service user (McLean *et al.* 2012). In order to achieve such understanding, it will therefore be necessary for you to recognise and work with the values of those who use mental health services and, while this can add a further dimension of complexity to your practice, it can also bring opportunities to move towards working in an increasingly person-centred, collaborative and empowering way with others.

Case study

Now in her late 20s, Kimberly became involved with mental health services while still a teenager. Following repeated instances of self-harm and a number of reported instances of 'challenging', 'disruptive' and 'inappropriate' behaviour, she was initially given a number of different diagnoses. Several years ago, however, she was informed that she was 'suffering from' borderline personality disorder (although she sometimes questions, argues about and even openly rejects that diagnosis). Although Kimberly has not been admitted to hospital for a while, she repeatedly presents to mental health services in a state of distress at varying times of the night and day. She often displays outbursts of anger and aggression, complaining of how people 'always let her down'; on other occasions she reports having feelings of intense sadness and guilt, believing that she is fundamentally 'weak', 'bad' or 'evil'. She sometimes says that she feels 'powerless' or that she is 'hollow inside' and periodically suggests that she feels as though she 'doesn't really exist'. Since the beginning of her involvement with mental health services she has continued to engage in self-harm behaviours; in particular, lacerating her forearms which, on occasion, has required medical intervention. For a number of years Kimberly has been prescribed and has been taking various antidepressants, but she states that these provide no benefit and that all she wants is someone 'genuine' to talk to, someone she can trust. Although she says that she can remember one or two staff members that she felt cared for her, people that she suggests provided her with 'security and comfort', she believes that the majority of staff now see her as a 'difficult' person, as someone who 'constantly pushes boundaries' and for whom very little can be done.

Activity 4.3	*Critical thinking*

For this activity, reflect upon Kimberly's experiences in the above case study and consider how values-based practice may influence your approach to working with her. In particular, consider the following questions:

continued . . .

- What does Kimberly appear to value at present?
- How might your personal values affect your mental health practice with Kimberly in both productive and potentially less productive ways?
- What professional values might be relevant when working with Kimberly?

An outline answer is provided at the end of the chapter.

Values and mental distress

The importance of recognising and working with personal values, professional values and the values of those who use mental health services will be a key aspect of your development towards becoming a self-aware, proactive and responsive mental health professional. However, critical discussions about the presence of values in contemporary mental health care extend beyond the recognition of the importance of practising in a values-based manner. One of the most enduring and significant of these discussions is concerned with the role that values play in understanding and conceptualising the experiences of those who use mental health services. Becoming aware of this critical discussion will not only enable you to develop deeper levels of critical thinking and critical reflection for your academic studies, but it will also enable you to think more critically about the assumptions, attitudes and beliefs that inform your own mental health practice.

Conceptualising mental distress

In order to begin to understand this critical discussion it is productive to note that arguably the most influential and enduring way of understanding and responding to mental distress, at least since the birth of psychiatry in the nineteenth century, has been to view it as the manifestation of a disease process that has a biological cause. The discipline that has been most closely associated with such an understanding is psychiatry and it is commonly suggested that psychiatry has sought to present itself as another branch of medicine, somewhat comparable to cardiology or neurology, that is concerned with diagnosing and treating people who are suffering from 'objectively' identifiable disorders that have an underlying biological basis (Ingleby 1981; Bentall 2004; Busfield 2011). This biological, or what is often referred to as the medical or biomedical model of mental distress, has profoundly influenced many aspects of mental health care; for example, it can be understood as manifesting itself in the language used to discuss mental distress (e.g. mental 'illness', 'patients' and 'symptoms'), the settings that are considered the most appropriate in which to provide mental health care (e.g. hospitals, wards and clinics) and the people who are deemed the most qualified to provide that care (e.g. doctors, nurses and other mental health 'clinicians'). In the context of thinking critically about the presence of values in contemporary mental health care, however, you should note that the biomedical model of mental distress is commonly thought of as being an objective, value-free and largely 'scientific' model of mental distress. Understood as a medical speciality that is comparable to cardiology or neurology, it has been suggested that psychiatry is concerned with presenting itself as identifying and treating 'naturally occurring' and therefore objective diseases in which personal, social and cultural value judgements supposedly play no part in the identification and treatment of those diseases (Boyle 2012; Johnstone 2014; Roberts 2014).

> ### Concept summary: Emil Kraepelin's 'big idea'
>
> One of the most influential figures in the development of a biological understanding of mental distress was the late nineteenth, early twentieth-century German psychiatrist, Emil Kraepelin. Kraepelin is often regarded as the 'father' of modern psychiatry, in part because of his introduction of two diagnostic categories: dementia praecox (later reformulated by Eugen Bleuler as schizophrenia) and manic-depressive insanity. However, it has also been suggested that his importance resides in the manner in which he introduced what has been referred to as his 'big idea', a new **paradigm** or way of thinking about mental distress (Ion & Beer 2002; Bentall 2004; Pilgrim 2007). In particular, Kraepelin's big idea consisted of making a number of assumptions that have profoundly influenced psychiatry and which include the following:
>
> - There are a number of separate and naturally occurring mental illnesses.
> - Each mental illness is characterised by a particular set of symptoms.
> - Each mental illness is caused by different types of brain disease.

Signs and symptoms

Against the supposedly objective, value-free character of psychiatry, however, it has been suggested that a variety of psychological, sociological and cultural value judgements are inherent in the identification of mental disorders (Szasz 1983; Watters 2011; Johnstone 2014). In order to begin to understand this, it will be productive for you to remember the common distinction that is made in health care between **signs** and **symptoms**. Symptoms are understood as referring to the subjective experiences and feelings that people often report to health care professionals – such as dizziness, stomach ache or nausea – whereas signs are the objective, physical indications of the potential presence of disease – such as a low white blood cell count, an irregular pulse rate or high blood pressure. While the identification of disease or disorder in any area of health care is a complex process, it has been suggested that, in order to do so in a valid and reliable way, both signs and symptoms are necessary (Boyle 2012). Although symptoms can provide the first indication of potential health care problems, they can be highly subjective and can have many possible causes; therefore, the presence of a disorder or a disease is identified when those symptoms are associated with the physical manifestation of the disease, with signs that can be objectively detected and verified by medical measures, such as blood tests, X-rays and tissue samples. It is important to note, however, that in contrast to the identification of diseases and disorders in other areas of health care there are, for the majority of cases, no signs by which the identification of 'mental illness' or 'mental disorder' can be made (Johnstone 2008; Barker 2009b). Rather, the identification and diagnosis of mental disorders such as schizophrenia, bipolar affective disorder and personality disorder are made on the basis of symptoms and, in particular, on the basis of judgements about the thoughts, feelings and behaviours of those people who come into contact with mental health services.

Case study

Laura is a first-year mental health nursing student who, having just returned from a visit to Kimberly with her mentor, is beginning to reflect critically upon the diagnosis of borderline personality disorder. As she discusses her reflections with Owen – a third-year mental health nursing student who is on the same clinical placement – he tells her that, of course, there are no physical tests that can establish a diagnosis of borderline personality disorder such as a blood test or a brain scan but the process is 'relatively straightforward'. In particular, he suggests that it involves observing if a person meets the criteria in, for example, the 'DSM' (APA 2013) or the 'ICD' (WHO 1992) by displaying symptoms such as 'impulsive behaviour', 'unstable personal relationships', 'inappropriate anger' or 'emotional instability'. Laura says she understand this, but wonders who defines what is to be considered 'inappropriate' anger or an 'unstable' relationship, and then begins to reflect upon why they should be seen as symptoms of a disorder or a disease at all when there are no tests to confirm this. Owen states that she is seeing a problem where there isn't one; however, although she is having difficulty clarifying her concerns, Laura still has a sense that there is something questionable about referring to someone's personality as 'disordered'.

Cultural value judgements

To the extent that the identification of mental disorder is made on the basis of symptoms without the support of signs, without being able to detect underlying biological pathology by medical investigations, then it has been suggested that psychiatry employs a variety of psychological, sociological and cultural value judgements; indeed, in relation to the attempt to classify mental disorders on the basis of symptoms, exemplified in the diagnostic systems referred to by Owen in the case study above, Bentall (2004, p. 139) has suggested that *this enterprise is, itself, culture bound. It represents the efforts of members of one particular culture to make sense of human behavioural breakdowns.* However, critically thinking about the role that cultural value judgements may play in the theoretical assumptions and the practical formulation of a psychiatric diagnosis can be a particular challenge, not least because of the manner in which the objective, value-free notion of such an activity is said to be interwoven with a number of fundamental interventions and powerful interest groups in contemporary mental health care (Moncrieff 2008; Johnstone 2014).

You may therefore find that a productive way to begin to think critically about the role of cultural value judgements in psychiatric diagnoses is, like Laura in the above case study, to consider critically a single psychiatric diagnosis such as the category of personality disorder. Indeed, it has been suggested that the category of personality disorder, perhaps more so than any other diagnostic category used in contemporary mental health care, discloses the value judgements that are employed in the identification of mental disorders (Crowe & Carlyle 2009; Cromby *et al.* 2013a). In particular, it is argued that in order to identify a person as having a disordered personality, then it is necessary to do so against the background of some notion of what it means to have an ordered or a normal personality; however, what constitutes an ordered or a normal personality is said to be dependent upon the values and the norms of a particular culture at a particular historical period, on a host of implicit and explicit value judgements about how people ought to think, feel and behave, such that no value-free distinction between an ordered and a disordered personality can be made (Gunn & Potter 2015).

Activity 4.4   *Evidence-based practice and research*

Emergence is a service-user-led organisation that provides information, advice and support for people affected by, or people caring for someone affected by, a diagnosis of personality disorder. For this activity, go to their website (**www.emergenceplus.org.uk**) and, in particular, read and consider the critical discussion entitled 'Why are personality disorders controversial diagnoses?'

As this activity is based on your own research, there is no outline answer at the end of the chapter.

Reconceptualising mental distress

It is important to recognise that, in suggesting that the identification of mental disorder is made on the basis of cultural value judgements about a person's thoughts, feelings and behaviours, this does not mean that the experiences of those who use mental health services should somehow be understood as being 'less credible' or 'less real' than in other areas of health care. As you will be aware, the experiences of those who use mental health services can be unusual, distressing and even profoundly disturbing, both for themselves and for others. However, the critical question that has been asked is whether those experiences should be presented as the manifestation of objective disorders or diseases with underlying physical causes when, in the majority of cases, psychiatric diagnoses are made exclusively on the basis of symptoms and, in particular, psychological, social and cultural value judgements about how people ought to think, feel and behave. As Johnstone (2013, p. 109) has suggested, *the problem arises when subjectivity is presented as objectivity, or to put it another way, when social and cultural judgements are presented as if they were medical ones about bodily problems.*

The significance of your critical thinking and reflection about this issue, and the presence of value judgements in the identification of mental disorders more generally, will not only be pertinent for your academic studies and the development of your capacity for critical thought and reflection. How you think about the sometimes distressing thoughts, feelings and behaviours of those who use mental health services will not only influence how you conceptualise mental distress, and your thoughts about how best to respond to that distress, but will also have significant consequences for those who use mental health services. For example, understanding mental distress as a disorder or a disease may provide those who use mental health services, along with those closest to them, with a ready explanation for their difficulties and may provide relief and reassurance as a result. However, it has been suggested that such an understanding can have a number of less productive consequences that can restrict and even prevent the establishment of therapeutic practices and recovery-orientated approaches to mental health care; in particular, it has variously been suggested that understanding mental distress as a disorder or a disease can place those experiencing such distress in the passive position of the **sick role**, that it can deprive such distress of any personal meaning for the individual and that it can lead to stigma and **discrimination**, the long-term consequences of which can be more damaging than the mental distress itself (Honos-Webb & Leitner 2001; Johnstone 2014). It has therefore been suggested that, rather than the symptoms of a disease, the thoughts, feelings and behaviours associated with mental distress may be better understood as responses to a whole range of 'problems in living' such as adverse circumstances, traumatic experiences and problematic interpersonal relationships; situated within the unique history and current context of each individual's life, the thoughts, feelings and behaviours associated with mental distress may be better understood as reactions to, and ways of making tolerable, what are experienced as profound psychological, sociological and even philosophical problems in living (Laing 1960; Szasz 1983; Boyle 2002; Bentall 2004).

Activity 4.5   *Team working*

It has been suggested that the thoughts, feelings and behaviours of those with a diagnosis of borderline personality disorder – rather than being seen as symptoms of a disease or a disorder – are understandable responses to adverse life events and strategies for coping with difficult circumstances and relationships. Consider Kimberly's thoughts, feelings and behaviours in the above case study and, with your colleagues, discuss how they might be understood as a response to, and ways of coping with, adverse life events and problems in living more generally.

An outline answer is provided at the end of the chapter.

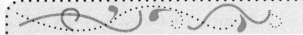

Chapter summary

In this chapter we have discussed the importance of values and the significance of values in contemporary mental health care. In doing so, the importance of critically thinking about, and critically reflecting upon, values has been set within the context of the therapeutic use of self and the ability to establish therapeutic relationships and supportive, enabling alliances with those who use mental health services. However, in addition to highlighting the importance of gaining an awareness of how personal values can affect your practice in both productive and non-productive ways, we have also considered whether mental health nursing has its own particular set of professional values. While gaining an awareness of personal and professional values will be central to your ability to establish supportive, therapeutic relationships with others, this chapter has also stressed the importance of being able to recognise and work with the values of those who use mental health services and it has done so within the context of values-based practice.

continued . . .

• •

Finally, this chapter has introduced you to one of the most enduring and significant critical discussions surrounding the role of values in contemporary mental health care and, in
particular, the role that values play in understanding, conceptualising and responding to
mental distress. In doing so, this chapter has not only sought to encourage you to develop
your critical thinking and reflection capabilities for your academic studies, but has also
encouraged you to think more critically about the assumptions, attitudes and values that
inform your own mental health nursing practice.

• •

Activities: brief outline answers

Activity 4.3 Critical thinking

Attempting to elicit a person's values can be a particular challenge and, to do so, you will need to develop
supportive, trusting relationships with those who use mental health services. However, from the information given in the case study, you may have identified how Kimberly appears to value relationships in which
she does not feel 'let down', relationships in which she feels she is able to 'trust' others and achieve a
degree of 'security'. You may also have suggested that she not only appears to value the importance of being
'genuine' but, from her reported feelings of powerlessness and possibly her disputes over her diagnosis,
the importance of establishing an element of control, **self-determination** and independence in her life. In
terms of your personal values, you may have identified a variety that could have a positive, productive
impact on your mental health nursing practice with Kimberly, including compassion, acceptance and
empathy; however, you may also have recognised that some of her thoughts, feelings and behaviours could
potentially conflict with your values and might elicit less positive and productive thoughts, feelings and
behaviours within you. Indeed, it has been suggested that negative attitudes and value judgements towards
those with a diagnosis of borderline personality disorder, and personality disorder more generally, are
prevalent among mental health professionals (Proctor 2007; Wright *et al.* 2007; Westwood & Baker 2010).
Finally, you may have identified a variety of professional values that are pertinent to your mental health
nursing practice with Kimberly, including the need to respond to her apparent personal values with the
professional values of compassion, genuineness and trust; in addition, you may have noted the relevance
of a variety of values that have been identified as being pertinent to contemporary mental health care, such
as combating stigma and exclusion, facilitating recovery and promoting safety and positive risk taking.

Activity 4.5 Team working

In attempting to determine how Kimberly's thoughts, feelings and behaviours might be understood as a
response to, and strategies for coping with, adverse life events – as opposed to being symptoms of a disorder
or a disease – then it will be necessary to situate her experiences in the unique context of her life. However,
while you ought to be cautious about making generalisations regarding those who use mental health services, it has been suggested that a significant number of people who are diagnosed with borderline personality disorder report having a history of experiencing childhood trauma such as emotional, sexual and
violent physical abuse (Castillo 2003). While it would be necessary to consider such findings in the context
of Kimberly's unique life history and current experience, you may have discussed with your colleagues the
possibility of how her displays of anger and aggression, her feelings of guilt and powerlessness and the
apparent value that she places on trust and security might be responses to previous experiences of trauma
and abuse. In addition, you may have had interesting discussions with your colleagues about how Kimberly's
repeated engagement in self-harm behaviours and her possible 'dissociative' experiences – reflected in her
sense of detachment and feeling as though she 'doesn't really exist' – may be understood as strategies to
combat feelings of powerlessness and achieve a degree of control and self-determination over her life
(Warner & Wilkins 2003; Proctor 2007).

Further reading

Fulford KWM, Peile E & Carroll H (2012) *Essential Values-Based Practice: Clinical stories linking science with people.* Cambridge: Cambridge University Press.

This is a comprehensive book that details the theory and practice of working in a values-based manner and how it can be understood as a complementary framework to evidence-based practice.

Johnstone L (2014) *A Straight Talking Introduction to Psychiatric Diagnosis.* Ross-on-Wye: PCCS Books.

An accessible introduction to contemporary critical debates surrounding psychiatric diagnosis which includes a discussion of its impact on those who use mental health services as well as alternatives to psychiatric diagnosis.

Szasz T (1983) The myth of mental illness, in Szasz T (ed) *Ideology and Insanity: Essays on the psychiatric dehumanization of man.* London: Marion Boyars.

Here you will find the classic critical discussion of the role that values play in the identification of mental illness by one of the most provocative and controversial figures in psychiatry.

Watters E (2011) *Crazy Like Us: The globalization of the Western mind.* London: Constable & Robinson.

This is a stimulating book that highlights the cultural values that are inherent in Western understandings of mental distress and, in particular, discusses how these are being 'exported' to other cultures around the world.

Useful websites

www.dxsummit.org

This is the website for the Global Summit on Diagnostic Alternatives (GSDA) and it provides an open forum for critiques of, and alternatives to, psychiatric diagnosis from a multiplicity of perspectives.

www.emergenceplus.org.uk

Here you will find the website for the service-user-led organisation called Emergence, which provides a variety of resources on personality disorder diagnoses, including an informative overview of the controversies surrounding those diagnoses.

Chapter 5
Others and difference

NMC Standards for Pre-registration Nursing Education

This chapter will address the following competencies:

Domain 1: Professional values

2   All nurses must practise in a holistic, non-judgemental, caring and sensitive manner that avoids assumptions; supports social inclusion; recognises and respects individual choice; and acknowledges diversity. Where necessary, they must challenge inequality, discrimination and exclusion from access to care.

3.1 Mental health nurses must promote mental health and wellbeing, while challenging the inequalities and discrimination that may arise from or contribute to mental health problems.

Domain 2: Communication and interpersonal skills

1   All nurses must build partnerships and therapeutic relationships through safe, effective and non-discriminatory communication. They must take account of individual differences, capabilities and needs.

Domain 3: Nursing practice and decision-making

1.1 Mental health nurses must be able to recognise and respond to the needs of all people who come into their care including babies, children and young people, pregnant and postnatal women, people with physical health problems, people with physical disabilities, people with learning disabilities, older people, and people with long-term problems such as cognitive impairment.

Chapter aims

By the end of this chapter you will be able to:

- identify the manner in which people who use mental health services are subject to stigma, discrimination and exclusion;
- describe how stigma, discrimination and exclusion affect different groups of mental health service users in different ways;
- understand the importance of developing a non-stigmatising, anti-discriminatory and socially inclusive mental health nursing practice.

Introduction

Case study

Almost ten years before becoming a mental health nurse, Samuel was given a diagnosis of bipolar affective disorder. He believes that his experience of mental distress provides him with valuable insights into what it is like to be a mental health service user and informs his work as a mental health nurse more generally. However, despite working within the mental health services, he feels unable to disclose his experience of mental distress to his colleagues and is concerned that they may discover his mental health history. He fears that if they knew then he would not only lose credibility as a mental health practitioner but would also be discredited as a person. Rather than being understood as an everyday, 'normal' display of emotion, for example, any expression of sadness, irritability, enthusiasm or happiness would potentially be seen as a symptom of a 'manic' or a 'depressive' episode. However supportive or well intentioned, he believes that many of his colleagues would never be able to see beyond his diagnosis and whatever he said or did would always be judged in the context of that diagnosis.

One of the most significant critical issues in contemporary mental health care concerns the manner in which those who experience, or have experienced, mental distress are affected by various forms of stigma, discrimination and exclusion. As you may already be aware, people with mental health problems have been found to be significantly disadvantaged in a number of ways, including having reduced employment and educational opportunities; having fewer supportive relationships and more limited social networks; being more likely to experience poverty and to live in poor localities; having higher rates of physical health problems; receiving poorer standards of physical health care; and having an increased risk of dying prematurely (Thornicroft 2006; Rogers & Pilgrim 2014). In order to become an informed, proactive and socially inclusive mental health practitioner, it will be necessary for you to begin to reflect critically upon, and to consider how to address, the manner in which such disadvantage and inequality can be understood as a consequence of stigma, **prejudice** and discrimination. In order to achieve this, you will be required to think critically about the underlying processes by which those people who experience mental distress can be subject to practices of exclusion and, more profoundly, can be physically and symbolically separated from the rest of society by being designated as 'different' or 'other'. However, an important critical concern about mental health services has also focused on the degree to which they have adequately recognised, respected and productively responded to the difference and diversity that characterise those who experience mental health difficulties and who use mental health services. Therefore, it will not only be necessary for you to gain an appreciation of the processes by which people with mental health difficulties are subject to practices of exclusion, but you will also be required to think critically about how stigma, prejudice and discrimination affect different groups of mental health service users in different ways and how you can begin to address such issues in your mental health nursing practice.

The purpose of this chapter is to introduce you to the manner in which those who experience mental distress have often been thought of as being different from the rest of society's members and, as a consequence of that difference, have been subject to stigma, prejudice and discrimination. It will begin by introducing you to the underlying processes by which certain groups of people – on the basis of particular behaviours, beliefs or experiences – are designated as different or 'other' and physically and symbolically separated from the rest of society. However, as well as discussing the general processes by which people with mental health difficulties are subject to practices of exclusion, this chapter will also introduce you to how stigma, prejudice and discrimination can be understood as affecting different groups of mental health service users in different ways. While there has been extensive critical debate about how different groups of people have significantly different experiences of mental health care, this chapter will look at three different groups in particular: first, it will introduce you to critical considerations about how the quality of mental health care received by individuals can be influenced by their gender; second, it will discuss how ethnicity can influence their experience of mental health services; finally, it will examine how people's experience of the quality of mental health care that they receive can be influenced by their age. By doing so, this chapter will not only encourage you to think critically about the processes by which different groups of people are said to be subject to practices of exclusion in contemporary mental health care, but will also encourage you to reflect critically upon how to develop as a non-stigmatising, anti-discriminatory and socially inclusive mental health practitioner.

The other

The processes by which people who experience mental distress are subject to stigma, discrimination and exclusion are both complex and multidimensional, and a variety of psychological, sociological and **anthropological** explanations have been proposed (Hinshaw 2010). However, it has been suggested that what underlies the manner in which any group of people – including those who experience mental distress – are subject to stigma, discrimination and exclusion is a process by which certain people are identified as being different from the rest of society's members and designated as 'other' (Said 1978; Foucault 2001; de Beauvoir 2015). It is important to recognise that the notion of 'the other' does not simply refer to other people but is used to designate those individuals who are seen as 'not belonging', as being 'outsiders' who possess characteristics and attributes that are not only different but that are judged to be unsatisfactory, undesirable and unwanted. Indeed, in the most extreme case, those individuals who are situated in the position of being 'other' can come to be seen as inferior, deficient, and so fundamentally different from the rest of society that they are no longer thought of as being 'fully human' (Goffman 1963; Link & Phelan 2001). While the manner in which particular groups of people are placed in the position of being 'other' can be understood as serving a number of psychological, sociological and political functions, one of its most significant is to establish a distinction between 'us and them'. In particular, it has been suggested that the creation of a distinction between 'us and them' clearly demarcates which individuals are to be understood as society's 'outsiders', or who belong to the 'outgroup', so that we are able to reassure ourselves that we are part of the 'ingroup'. As Littlewood and Lipsedge (1997, p. 27) have suggested, *We forget that the outsiders are part of our definition of ourselves. To confirm our own identity we push the outsiders even further away. By reducing their humanity we emphasize our own.*

Activity 5.1   *Evidence-based practice and research*

It is commonly suggested that one of the most powerful influences on positioning those who experience mental distress as 'other' and, by doing so, establishing a distinction between 'us and them', is the **mass media**. A significant amount of research has indicated that the mass media perpetuates negative, false and **stereotypical** images of mental distress, variously representing those people who experience mental health difficulties as violent, unpredictable, dependent and childlike (Henderson 2008; Walsh 2009; Philo *et al.* 2010).

Over the next two weeks, take note of any instances of mental distress being represented and reported in the mass media such as on television, in films and in newspapers and magazines.

- Do those representations perpetuate what you think is a negative stereotypical image of mental distress?
- Do those representations present what you think is a positive, more inclusive image of mental distress?

As this activity is based on your own research, there is no outline answer at the end of the chapter.

It is important to recognise that the manner in which those who experience mental distress are positioned as being 'other', along with the establishment of a distinction between 'us and them', can be a consequence of the activities of large entities and organisations such as the mass media. However, it is equally important to recognise that the creation of a distinction between 'us and them' through the perpetuation of stereotypical images, the assertion of sweeping generalisations and the employment of exclusionary language can also be a feature of the everyday activities of individual health care practitioners. For example, while many mental health professionals work in productive ways to challenge stigma, prejudice and exclusion, it has been suggested that mental health professionals can perpetuate negative, discriminatory attitudes towards those who use mental health services and, in doing so, can establish and maintain the distinction between 'us and them' (Wright *et al.* 2007; Ross & Goldner 2009).

Case study

Midway through their night shift on an acute mental health ward, Gina and Elliot are discussing a mental health service user who was admitted earlier that evening with a history of substance use problems. Gina states that she is becoming frustrated by the amount of 'users' that are increasingly being admitted on to the ward and doesn't understand why they are treated by mental health services. Elliot says he shares Gina's frustration and adds that those who use drugs and alcohol are increasingly becoming a 'drain' on the limited resources of mental health services: all that time and energy is spent

continued . . .

on getting them 'clean' and as soon as they are discharged from hospital they start using again. Gina agrees and suggests that there's 'next to nothing' that can be done for them and mental health services would be better off caring for those who have 'genuine' mental health problems.

In order to develop your non-stigmatising, anti-discriminatory and socially inclusive mental health nursing practice, it will be important for you to begin to recognise, critically reflect upon and actively challenge simplistic generalisations, stereotypical assumptions and the employment of exclusionary language – all of which can arguably be evidenced in the above case study. Indeed, it has been suggested that mental health nursing students are in a particularly valuable position to become aware of, and to reflect critically upon, the negative attitudes, generalisations and stereotypes that can contribute to a distinction between 'us and them' in contemporary mental health care (Maccallum 2002). While you may be eager to qualify as a mental health nurse, your position as a mental health nursing student can be understood as a valuable one insofar as it can enable you to bring a fresh, critical perspective to contemporary mental health services and discern the presence of potentially discriminatory practices that may go unnoticed by more established and experienced practitioners. In particular, it can enable you to reflect critically upon the potential positioning of those who use mental health services as different or 'other', to think critically about how and why the establishment of a distinction between 'us and them' occurs and, finally, to begin to consider critically how you might go about seeking to question, challenge and change the potential presence of such a distinction in contemporary mental health care.

Difference

Although stigma, discrimination and exclusion can be understood as involving a positioning of people who experience mental distress as different or 'other', an enduring criticism of mental health services has been that they have not adequately recognised, respected and productively responded to the difference and diversity that characterise those who experience mental distress and who use mental health services. In particular, it has been suggested that a common tendency associated with the positioning of any group as 'other' is to perceive the members of that group as **homogeneous**, as sharing common characteristics and lacking differentiation (Ben-Zeev *et al.* 2010). In order to resist such a tendency in your mental health nursing practice, it will be necessary to begin to recognise, and critically reflect upon, how stigma, discrimination and exclusion affect different groups of mental health service users in different ways. For the remainder of the chapter we shall therefore discuss how individuals' experiences of mental health services can be influenced by a variety of factors and, in particular, by their gender, ethnicity and age. However, it is important to recognise that an individual's experience of mental health services may not only be affected by any combination of these three factors, but may also be affected by a variety of other factors, including sexuality, socio-economic status, spirituality and disability. The challenge facing you as you progress through your mental health nursing programme is to begin to recognise the multiplicity of factors that may be influencing your clinical encounters with those who use contemporary mental health services, and to think critically about how to respond in a manner that reflects non-stigmatising, anti-discriminatory and socially inclusive mental health nursing practice.

Gender

Case study

As part of the third-year Professional Issues in Mental Health Nursing module, Adriana is reviewing her portfolio of learning that she has kept over the duration of her mental health nursing course. In doing so, she notices that the majority of her reflective pieces over the three years have been about her experiences of working with female mental health service users. As she reflects on those experiences more deeply, and the variety of clinical settings in which those experiences occurred, she becomes aware that in most of those settings there seemed to be more female service users than men. She is a little surprised that she had never noticed this before and begins to wonder if the apparent presence of more female mental health service users is simply a reflection of her experience or if it is perhaps a feature of mental health services more generally.

One of the most enduring and contested critical issues in contemporary mental health care concerns gender and, in particular, the extent to which being a man or a woman influences an individual's experience of mental distress and the quality of mental health care received as a response to that distress. For example, critical discussions exist about the seemingly different forms of mental distress that are experienced by men and women, the different ways in which men and women report mental distress and access mental health services and the different treatment and interventions that men and women receive from mental health professionals (Coppock 2008). However, the one gender issue that has been the subject of extensive critical debate – and which Adriana is beginning to reflect upon critically in the above case study – is the degree to which, overall, women receive a psychiatric diagnosis more often than men and are more likely to have been treated for a mental health problem (Rogers & Pilgrim 2014).

While a variety of explanations for this have been proposed – such as making reference to the research which indicates that women are more likely to seek professional help for mental distress than men – one of the most enduring critical explanations is that the over-representation of women in psychiatric diagnosis is a reflection of gender stereotypes and assumptions. In particular, it has been suggested that mental health professionals hold differing expectations about what attitudes and behaviours are appropriate for women compared with men such that women are more likely to be given a psychiatric diagnosis if they deviate too far from what is considered 'appropriate feminine behaviour' (Chesler 1972; Showalter 1987; Ussher 1991). For example, it has been suggested that the high incidence of women with a diagnosis of borderline personality disorder is to be understood as a consequence of a gender bias maintained by mental health professionals; in particular, it has been argued that displays of anger, aggression and 'impulsivity' – understood as including 'reckless' driving, multiple sexual partners and gambling (APA 2013) – are more likely to be seen as symptomatic of a mental disorder in women than men because those behaviours are perceived by mental health professionals as not being in accordance with behaviour that is considered 'normal', 'appropriate' and 'acceptable' for women (Potter 2007; Proctor 2007).

Activity 5.2   *Critical thinking*

An alternative explanation for the over-representation of women in psychiatric diagnosis suggests that women are subject to particular demands, pressures and social disadvantage that make them more vulnerable to mental distress than men.

- What particular expectations may be placed on women, and what everyday stressors might they be subject to, that might contribute to higher rates of mental distress for women?

An outline answer is provided at the end of the chapter.

While extensive critical debate about the role of gender in contemporary mental health care services has focused on the experiences of women, and the over-representation of women in psychiatric diagnosis in particular, it is important to recognise the impact of gender expectations, assumptions and stereotyping on men. For example, it has been suggested that men are less likely to acknowledge and seek help for certain types of mental distress, such as depression, anxiety and eating disorders, because such distress is seen as being characteristically 'feminine' and therefore incompatible with traditional notions of 'masculinity' (Doherty & Kartalova-O'Doherty 2010; Strother *et al.* 2012). In particular, the traditional gender role expectation that men should be independent, controlled and self-sufficient is said potentially to inhibit the acknowledgement of mental distress by men insofar as seeking help may be understood as admitting an inability to handle things on one's own. As a consequence, it has been suggested that men are more likely to rely on themselves, to withdraw socially or to employ their own coping strategies, such as using drugs and alcohol, to alleviate the experience of mental distress (Courtenay 2000). As we have suggested, a fundamental aspect of critical thinking and critical reflection in mental health nursing is the ability to identify the assumptions, values and beliefs that are governing our thoughts, feelings and actions in a given situation. As an aspect of this, it will therefore be important for you to think critically about the gender expectations, assumptions and potential stereotypes that may be influencing your mental health practice. In particular, it will be necessary to consider critically how your gender expectations and assumptions may be influencing how you understand and respond to the mental distress of men and women differently and, where necessary, how you might go about challenging and changing those expectations in order to provide mental health care that does not stigmatise, discriminate or exclude on the basis of gender.

Ethnicity

The treatment and experiences of people from black and minority ethnic communities by mental health services is one of the most controversial critical issues in contemporary mental health care. Before discussing this issue, however, it is first important to recognise that the identification of people on the basis of ethnicity can itself be a complex and disputed procedure, not least because ethnic identification is multidimensional, dynamic and self-defined and incorporates a variety of elements, including language, religion, spirituality, nationality and a person's ancestral place of origin.

While noting the complexity of ethnic identification, however, black and minority ethnic communities are commonly understood as referring to people with black African, African Caribbean, South Asian and Chinese heritage, as well as including people from the Irish community and Eastern European communities (Pelle 2014). While these groups are collectively referred to as black and minority ethnic communities, this does not imply that those communities are a single, homogeneous group; rather, it is important to recognise that a multiplicity of differences will exist both within and between those communities. However, it has been suggested that, when taken as a collective, what is common across these communities is that they experience significant inequalities in mental health care when compared with the majority white community.

In particular, people from black and minority ethnic communities are more likely to be compulsorily admitted to mental health services, to be treated in a secure setting and to be subject to 'coercive practices' such as seclusion and physical restraint; there is an increased likelihood that people from those communities will also be prescribed medication and electroconvulsive therapy, rather than receiving psychological interventions such as psychotherapy and counselling; in addition, it has been suggested that people from black and minority ethnic communities are more likely to have their mental distress misunderstood and misdiagnosed, while people from African Caribbean communities in particular are more likely to be perceived as violent and dangerous and to be given a diagnosis of schizophrenia (NIMHE 2003; JCPMH 2014; Rogers & Pilgrim 2014). A number of explanations for these inequalities have been given, including the impact of cultural differences, the increased social and economic disadvantage experienced by black and minority ethnic communities and the psychological stress surrounding migration and **acculturation**. However, one of the most contentious explanations for ethnic inequalities in mental health care has been the accusation of racial prejudice and, in particular, the suggestion that mental health services are 'institutionally racist' (Fernando 2008).

Concept summary: Institutional racism in mental health services

On 30 October 1998, David Bennett, a 38-year-old African Caribbean mental health service user with a diagnosis of schizophrenia, died in a medium-secure mental health unit after being physically restrained by staff. As part of its investigations into David Bennett's death, the subsequent inquiry by Norfolk, Suffolk & Cambridgeshire Strategic Health Authority (2003, p. 25) suggested that *institutional racism has been present in the mental health services, both NHS and private, for many years*. In doing so, it employed a definition of **institutional racism** that had been formulated by the Stephen Lawrence Inquiry four years earlier (Macpherson 1999, ¶6.34) in which institutional racism was defined as:

> *The collective failure of an organisation to provide an appropriate and professional service to people because of their colour, culture, or ethnic origin. It can be seen or detected in processes, attitudes and behaviour which amount to discrimination through unwitting prejudice, ignorance, thoughtlessness and racist stereotyping which disadvantage minority ethnic people.*

(Continued)

(Continued)

In expanding upon this definition, the Stephen Lawrence Inquiry proposed that institutional racism can persist and prevail as part of an organisation's ethos or culture when that organisation fails to recognise and address racism openly and adequately through anti-racist policies, training and leadership (Macpherson 1999, ¶6.34). In addition, the inquiry into David Bennett's death highlighted that a popular and serious misconception about institutional racism is that it is deliberate, whereas the inquiry stressed that prejudice and discrimination could occur through the unreflective, thoughtless and unwitting perpetuation of racist assumptions and stereotypes (Norfolk, Suffolk & Cambridgeshire Strategic Health Authority 2003, p. 43).

The suggestion that mental health services are institutionally racist is a controversial, challenging and complex one that has been the subject of ongoing critical discussion (McKenzie & Bhui 2007; Patel & Heginbotham 2007; Fernando 2010). However, partly as a response to the accusation of institutional racism in mental health services, and partly as a response to the inequalities experienced by black and minority ethnic communities in those services, there has been an increased focus on the need to provide culturally sensitive, competent and capable mental health care. As you progress through your mental health nursing programme, it will therefore be important for you not only to begin to gain an awareness of, and develop a respect for, the traditions, beliefs and value systems of people from black and minority ethnic communities, but also to reflect critically upon how your own ethnic and cultural identity affects your mental health practice. However, it is also important to recognise that, because of the potentially broad ethnic diversity of those people who use mental health services, then it may not be possible for you to understand all of the possible cultural influences that both you and mental health service users bring to the clinical encounter (O'Brien *et al.* 2009). Despite this, it will be possible for you to practise in such a way that you provide opportunities for all people who use mental health services to make their cultural needs known; while this will require the employment of a variety of skills, attributes and capabilities, it will be important for you to begin to develop, and to seek to maintain the development of, your capability to engage in effective cross-cultural communication and the provision of culturally competent mental health care more generally (Pelle 2014).

Activity 5.3   *Reflection*

The need for contemporary mental health services to provide culturally sensitive, competent and capable mental health care has repeatedly been affirmed. However, it has also been suggested that cultural competence and capability training in health care education programmes, and the presence of culturally capable practice in health care environments more generally, has been inconsistent at best (Holland & Hogg 2010).

For this activity, reflect upon your experience of the issue of culturally capable care being discussed in the academic setting and your experience of witnessing the provision of culturally capable care in the clinical environment.

continued . . .

- What teaching, training or information have you received about culturally capable mental health care?
- What evidence have you seen of culturally capable mental health care being provided in the clinical environment?
- How prepared do you feel to provide culturally capable mental health care?

As this activity is based on your own reflections, there is no outline answer at the end of the chapter.

Age

In addition to gender and ethnicity, there has been increased critical consideration of the manner in which those who use mental health services experience stigma, discrimination and exclusion on the basis of age. For example, it has recently been suggested that mental health professionals have not only failed to recognise adequately the complex contemporary pressures that children and young people confront, but that there are also serious problems with children's and adolescents' mental health services, from prevention and early intervention through to inpatient services for vulnerable young people (Health Committee 2014). In particular, it has been claimed that young people with mental health difficulties not only experience negative attitudes and exclusionary practices from their peers, but that they may also be subject to unproductive responses from health care professionals who may downplay, or even be explicitly dismissive of, the reality of their difficulties (Rose *et al.* 2007; Young Minds 2010). Despite the recent concern about children's and young people's experience of contemporary mental health services, a significant amount of critical work has focused on the quality of mental health care received by 'older people'; however, it is important to recognise that the notion of 'older people', like the notion of gender and ethnicity, is itself a matter of critical discussion. While it is generally understood in chronological terms as referring to a person over the age of 65 years, there is no general agreement about the age at which an individual becomes an 'older person' and traditional, enduring definitions are rapidly changing for a variety of reasons. For example, healthier lifestyles, changes in the age of retirement, potentially greater material resources and advances in medicine are meaning that significant numbers of people have increased opportunities to maintain their physical and mental wellbeing for longer as they progress into later life such that an individual who is over 65 may not perceive him/herself as an 'older person' or accept being understood as such (Biggs *et al.* 2007).

Case study

Maxine and Alistair are at the beginning of their mental health nursing programme and are discussing which area of mental health care they would like to work in when they qualify. Maxine is uncertain but suggests that she might like to work in an acute mental health setting or could possibly see herself

continued . . .

> *working in forensic mental health services. In contrast, Alistair says that he would like to work in older adult mental health services and is almost certain that he would like to work with people with dementia. Maxine is a little surprised by this: she finds it difficult to understand why anyone would want to work with older adults, especially those with dementia, and suggests that it must be a 'depressing' area to work in. Alistair explains that he worked in that area as a mental health care assistant before starting his mental health nursing course and, while he found it challenging at times, he also found it to be especially rewarding. Maxine appreciates this but suggests that she has always found older people difficult to talk to, partly because she has nothing in common with them and partly because she has often found them to be 'a little repetitive, irritable and impatient'.*

While recognising the complexity of the notion of 'older people', and the diversity of capabilities and needs that can exist within that group, it has been suggested that people over the age of 65 have been subject to various forms of discrimination and exclusion from mental health services. For example, it has been argued that mental health policy and practice have historically been concerned with the needs of people below the age of 65, while even contemporary discussions and practice initiatives surrounding the notion of recovery have largely been conducted with minimal consideration of their application in the context of older adult mental health care (Adams & Collier 2009; Anderson 2011). Although the mental health needs of people over the age of 65 can be understood as receiving increased consideration through the introduction of, for example, the National Dementia Strategy (DH 2009), it has been suggested that contemporary mental health services are skewed towards providing dementia care and are inadequately responding to the range of mental health problems experienced by older people, including depression, anxiety and substance use problems (Rogers & Pilgrim 2014). However, in addition to discrimination and exclusion towards older people at the organisational and policy level, it has also been suggested that a variety of negative attitudes, simplistic generalisations and stereotypical assumptions are maintained about older people at the everyday practice level and, as in the case study above, expressed by individual mental health practitioners. In particular, older people with mental health problems not only confront the stigma that can be associated with mental distress but can also be subject to the common misconception that the occurrence of mental health problems in later life is inevitable; that is, it has been suggested that mental health professionals, and health care professionals more generally, often understand mental health problems such as depression and dementia to be a natural part of ageing and that the associated distress is something that older people simply have to accept (Beecham *et al.* 2008).

Activity 5.4   *Team working*

As the post Second World War generation, the so-called 'baby boomers', progress into later life, it has been suggested that our understanding, assumptions and attitudes towards older people will have to undergo a significant shift (Mental Health Foundation 2009). This generation has been characterised as having significantly different values, experiences and expectations in comparison to previous generations, including the expectation

continued . . .

of a significantly longer and healthier life than their parents and grandparents. In addition, this generation have the experience of living through a period of increased **individualism**, **liberalism** and **consumerism** and many were engaged in securing and supporting rights and recognition on issues surrounding gender, race and sexual orientation. As a consequence, it has been suggested that the post Second World War generation are not only more likely to display a critical, questioning disposition towards established authorities but are also more likely to possess an increased awareness of, and uncompromising attitude towards, their rights as citizens and consumers.

- What potential challenges might the post Second World War generation present to mental health services as they progress into later life?
- How might mental health services have to change as a result of that challenge?

An outline answer is provided at the end of the chapter.

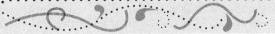

Chapter summary

In this chapter we have discussed how those who experience mental distress have often been thought of as being different from the rest of society's members and, as a consequence of that difference, have been subject to stigma, discrimination and exclusion. While the processes by which this occurs are complex, it has been suggested that underlying the manner in which those who experience mental distress are subject to practices of exclusion is the positioning of those people as different or 'other', a process which serves to establish a distinction between 'us and them' and clearly demarcates which individuals are to be understood as society's 'outsiders'. However, we have also critically examined the manner in which stigma, discrimination and exclusion affect different groups of mental health service users in different ways and, in particular, we have looked at how the quality of mental health care received by individuals can be influenced by their gender, their ethnicity and their age. In doing so, this chapter has encouraged you to begin to reflect critically upon the manner in which your assumptions, values and beliefs about gender, ethnicity and age may be negatively impacting upon how you understand and respond to those who use mental health services. Finally, it has also sought to encourage you, where necessary, to think critically about how you might begin to challenge and change those assumptions, values and beliefs in order to begin to develop your non-stigmatising, anti-discriminatory and socially inclusive mental health practice.

Activities: brief outline answers

Activity 5.2 Critical thinking

It has been suggested that there are a variety of expectations placed on women, and there are a number of everyday stressors that they are subject to, that may contribute to higher rates of mental distress for women when compared with men. In particular, it has been suggested that women are more likely to bear the greater burden of care responsibilities for children or significant others, such as parents or siblings; they are more likely to be economically dependent on others, to experience isolation in the home and be subject to domestic violence and sexual abuse; they are commonly subject to greater social pressures about their weight and appearance then men and, finally, for those women who do work outside the home, they are more likely to have low-paid, low-status jobs that restrict access to the resources that promote good mental health (Johnstone 2000).

Activity 5.4 Team working

Attempting to determine how the changing values, experiences and expectations of the post Second World War generation will challenge mental health services, and how those services may have to change as a result, is a particularly complex question. However, from the information given you may have had interesting discussions with your colleagues about how that generation, as they progress into later life, will have higher expectations of mental health services and will be more assertive users of those services. In particular, you may have discussed how they may be less deferential to mental health professionals and, as a result, how those professionals will increasingly need to work towards developing genuine collaborative relationships with older adults and respond to their demands for active involvement in older adult mental health services. Insofar as some members of the post Second World War generation were young at a time of increased availability and more liberal use of illegal drugs and alcohol, it has been suggested that mental health services may experience an increase in the numbers of older adults with substance use problems and, in doing so, they will have to take into account older substance users who may also have complex physical health care needs (Mental Health Foundation 2009). You may also have discussed how the creation of new specialist mental health services might be required that offer support for people who are active and still employed over the age of 65 but who are experiencing mental health problems such as depression, anxiety and substance use problems. In doing so, you may have identified the need for such services to be staffed by mental health professionals who are closer in age, life experience and general outlook to the service users with whom they are working and who may be more able to relate to the particular issues and mental health difficulties that the post Second World War generation may be experiencing.

Further reading

Fernando S (2010) *Mental Health, Race and Culture*, 3rd edition. Basingstoke: Palgrave Macmillan.

A comprehensive account of the impact of race and culture on contemporary mental health practice which includes, among other things, a critical discussion about the existence of racism in psychiatry.

Foucault M (2001) *Madness and Civilization: A history of insanity in the age of reason.* London: Routledge.

This is one of the most important, challenging and stimulating critical accounts of the contemporary understanding of mental distress that details how practices of exclusion emerged as a consequence of the historical construction of a distinction between reason and non-reason.

Goffman E (1963) *Stigma: Notes on the management of a spoiled identity.* Englewood Cliffs, NJ: Prentice-Hall.

Here you will find the classic discussion of the notion of stigma in which, through the extensive employment of autobiographies and case studies, the impact of stigma on the lives of individuals is examined.

Ussher JM (1991) *Women's Madness: Misogyny or mental illness?* Hemel Hempstead: Harvester Wheatsheaf.

This is a provocative account of women's experience of mental distress that discusses how gender expectations contribute to the identification of women as 'mad' and how this serves to silence their legitimate anger over social disadvantage and inequality.

Useful websites

www.ageuk.org.uk

Here you will find the website for Age UK, which provides a variety of resources, information and services that are designed to inspire, enable and support older people to make the most of later life.

www.time-to-change.org.uk

This is the website for the anti-stigma campaign led by the leading mental health charities Mind and Rethink Mental Illness; it aims to tackle the stigma, prejudice and discrimination surrounding mental distress.

Chapter 6
Interventions and involvement

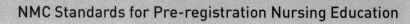
Chapter aims

By the end of this chapter you will be able to:

- identify a range of critical issues surrounding the use of psychiatric medication and psychological interventions in contemporary mental health care;
- understand a range of critical issues surrounding service user involvement and recovery-focused approaches in contemporary mental health care;
- reflect upon the implications of these critical issues for contemporary mental health nursing practice.

Introduction

Case study

As part of this week's tutorial for the Critical Perspectives in Mental Health Nursing module, Anisha, Claudia and Gareth have been asked to think critically about the range of interventions that are used in contemporary mental health care. In particular, they have been set the task of considering if there are any 'problematic' or 'contentious' issues surrounding any of those interventions and, if they think that there are, to express clearly what those concerns are. Although they have acknowledged that electro-convulsive therapy (ECT) remains a controversial intervention – and while they have all suggested that harsh and even brutal interventions were employed to respond to mental distress in the past – Anisha and her colleagues are finding it a challenge to identify anything contentious about the interventions that are used in contemporary mental health care. Indeed, they have all agreed that the interventions that are employed in contemporary mental health care are increasingly evidence-based and, within the context of service user involvement, person-centred care and recovery-focused practice, those who use mental health services are increasingly involved in decisions about the care and the interventions that they receive.

A wide variety of interventions exist in contemporary mental health care that are designed to limit, relieve or remove the suffering associated with mental distress. In order to begin to comprehend the diversity of interventions that are used, a general distinction is often made between physical interventions such as psychiatric medication, and psychological interventions such as counselling and psychotherapy. However, while the employment of both physical and psychological interventions to respond to mental distress is characteristic of contemporary mental health care, it is important to recognise that there also exists a variety of critical debates surrounding the theoretical assumptions and the practical employment of those interventions. While such debates have often been conducted by academics, researchers and mental health professionals, those people who use mental health services are increasingly calling into question the purpose, effectiveness and legitimacy of the physical and psychological interventions that are used to respond to mental distress. Indeed, the increasing involvement of mental health service users in the provision, evaluation and development of those services has, in recent years, emerged as one of the most significant features of contemporary mental health care. As well as the increased participation and collective action of service user groups in mental health services, the involvement of people who have had direct experience of mental distress has been a significant factor in the reorientation of mental health services towards recovery-focused principles and practice. However, despite the recovery-focused reorientation of mental health services, and the increased involvement of user groups in various aspects of those services, there exists a variety of critical considerations surrounding the notions of recovery and service user involvement that can be understood as having direct implications for your practice as a mental health nurse.

The purpose of this chapter is to introduce you to the various critical debates that surround the interventions used in contemporary mental health care and the involvement of those people who use mental health services in that care. While a number of physical interventions are used to respond to mental distress, and while you may already be aware of the controversy that surrounds some physical interventions such as ECT, we shall begin by discussing psychiatric medication insofar as it is the physical intervention that you are most likely to provide on a regular basis as a qualified mental health nurse. Similarly, while the formal provision of psychological therapies may not be part of your initial role as a mental health practitioner, mental health nurses do employ a wide range of counselling and psychotherapeutic skills in their everyday practice and this chapter will therefore introduce you to the critical issues surrounding the use of psychological interventions. We shall then examine the debates that have been concerned with the involvement of those people who use mental health services in the provision, evaluation and improvement of those services and, in particular, critical questions about the extent to which that involvement can be understood as 'genuine' or 'meaningful'. Finally, this chapter will introduce you to the critical issues that surround the notion of recovery and the extent to which a recovery-orientated approach can be reconciled with the range of responsibilities that mental health services are expected to meet, and the variety of roles that you are expected to perform as a responsible, proactive and accountable mental health practitioner.

Psychiatric medication

The use of medication as an intervention to respond to mental distress is central to contemporary mental health services and it continues to be the intervention that people who use those services are most likely to receive (Rogers & Pilgrim 2014). As a reflection of this, a notable period of your mental health nursing programme will be concerned with preparing you to be able to provide this intervention in a safe and competent manner. For example, in both the academic and the clinical setting, you will learn about the different classes of drugs used in psychiatry and their differing effects; you will be required to gain knowledge of, and practise in accordance with, established guidelines, procedures and standards for the safe storage and administration of medicines; finally, in preparation for registration as a qualified mental health nurse, you will be regularly observed dispensing medicines under supervision and your proficiency in doing so will be formally assessed. However, despite the centrality of psychiatric medication as a response to mental distress in contemporary mental health services, and despite the reported effectiveness of psychiatric drugs from a variety of sources, there exists a number of critical debates surrounding this form of intervention. For example, you are probably already aware that psychiatric medication can have a range of negative, adverse effects and there have been extensive critical discussions about the degree to which those effects outweigh the potential benefits of psychiatric drugs, and the extent to which those who take psychiatric medication are informed about, and actively involved in, those discussions; there are also critical concerns about how psychiatric medication is employed in the clinical setting and, in particular, concerns about various practices such as over-prescribing, **polypharmacy** and the use of excessive or 'mega-doses' of certain classes of psychiatric drugs; in addition, there are complex critical considerations about the quality of the research into the efficacy of psychiatric medication and, in particular, provocative analyses of the role of the pharmaceutical industry in this research and their influence upon mental health services more generally (Breggin 1993; Moncrieff 2008; Bentall 2010; Gøtzsche 2013).

Case study

Jonathan is in the fifth week of his clinical placement on a forensic mental health unit and his mentor, Celia, is providing him with feedback about his knowledge of psychiatric medication. Celia is particularly impressed with Jonathan's knowledge of both the generic and the trade names for common drugs used in psychiatry and also to which class each of those individual drugs belong. However, Jonathan is keen to deepen his knowledge about all aspects of psychiatric medication and asks his mentor how psychiatric drugs work. Celia replies that they work by acting upon the specific chemical imbalances and biological dysfunctions that are associated with mental distress and which give rise to the particular psychiatric symptoms that people experience. She goes on to suggest that how psychiatric drugs work is reflected in the names that are used to classify those drugs; so, for example, the drugs that target the chemical imbalances that lead to depression are called 'anti-depressants', the drugs that correct the biological mechanisms that cause psychosis are called 'anti-psychotics' and the drugs that act upon the underlying dysfunctions that lead to mood instability are called 'mood stabilisers'.

While there exists a number of critical debates surrounding psychiatric medication that focus variously on their effectiveness, their properties and their clinical use, one of the most fundamental critical discussions about psychiatric drugs is concerned with how they work. In the case study above, Jonathan's mentor is expressing the widely held explanation, sometimes referred to as the **disease-centred model**, that proposes that psychiatric drugs work by targeting specific underlying disease processes, somewhat similar to how insulin works in diabetes by compensating for the body's inability to produce sufficient quantities of that hormone. However, insofar as it has been suggested that there are problematic theoretical assumptions about the disease-centred model of psychiatric medication, along with methodological problems with the suggested evidence base for such an explanation, an alternative **drug-centred model** has been proposed (Moncrieff 2008; Moncrieff *et al.* 2013). In contrast to the disease-centred model, the drug-centred model of psychiatric medication suggests that psychiatric drugs do not work in a specific way by targeting underlying biological abnormalities or chemical imbalances; rather, the drug-centred model stresses that psychiatric drugs are psychoactive substances that act on the central nervous system to produce a range of altered mental and physical states that can not only produce adverse effects but may also produce effects that can alleviate the symptoms associated with mental distress. As Moncrieff (2013, p. 161) proposes, *The drug-centred model suggests that drugs can sometimes be helpful because the features of the altered drug-induced state superimpose themselves onto the manifestations of distress.* A common example of the drug-centred functioning of psychoactive substances is illustrated by some people's use of alcohol to relieve a range of symptoms associated with various forms of mental distress such as depression, anxiety and social phobias. In doing so, alcohol is not understood in a disease-centred way as targeting specific underlying biological dysfunctions or chemical imbalances; rather, it is understood in a drug-centred way as producing a range of altered mental and physical states (such as sedation, euphoria and disinhibition) that a person may temporarily experience as alleviating the physical and psychological symptoms associated with various forms of mental distress.

Activity 6.1   *Critical thinking*

As a qualified mental health nurse, there is an expectation that you will be involved in assisting those who use mental health services to make informed choices about psychiatric medication by providing education and information about their potential benefits and adverse effects and the possibility of alternative interventions (NMC 2010). However, it has been suggested that understanding psychiatric medication in terms of the disease-centred model can lead mental health professionals to minimise the potentially adverse effects of psychiatric drugs and the active involvement of mental health service users in discussions about the effects of, and alternatives to, those drugs (Moncrieff & Cohen 2009). That is, insofar as psychiatric drugs are understood as targeting specific underlying disease processes, then any negative consequences are presented as 'side effects' that, while potentially unpleasant, should not detract from the drug's supposedly 'main effects' of correcting the underlying biological dysfunction associated with mental distress.

- In contrast to the disease-centred model, how might the drug-centred model of psychiatric medication influence your discussions of the potential benefits, adverse effects and alternatives to psychiatric drugs with those who use mental health services?

An outline answer is provided at the end of the chapter.

Psychological interventions

Although psychiatric medication continues to be the dominant intervention in contemporary mental health care, those who use mental health services frequently voice a preference for psychological interventions and, partly as a response to this, there has been a commitment to increase access to a range of psychological therapies (DH 2014). Although you may not receive training in psychological therapies as part of your mental health nursing programme, and while the formal provision of those therapies may not be part of your initial role as a newly qualified mental health nurse, you will become increasingly aware that mental health nurses employ a wide range of counselling skills and psychotherapeutic techniques in their everyday practice. Indeed, being uniquely positioned to do so, it has been suggested that mental health nurses should continue to develop their ability to incorporate such skills into their daily practice, and many undertake supplementary training in order to enable them to deliver a variety of psychological therapies and psychosocial interventions (Winship & Hardy 2014; Walker 2015).

Despite the generally expressed preference of mental health service users for psychological therapies, and the continued commitment to increase the provision of a range of psychological interventions, there has been ongoing critical debate about those interventions from a variety of perspectives. For example, there are complex critical discussions about the quality of the research into, and the evidence base for, the therapeutic effectiveness of psychological therapies; there are also critical examinations of the manner in which psychological interventions are employed in the clinical setting and, in particular, challenging considerations about trust, the imbalance of power and various forms of exploitation in psychotherapy; more generally, there exist sociological, political and philosophical critiques that question the apparent expansion of a 'therapeutic, confessional culture' into widening areas of our lives, as well as critical questions about the function of individual psychotherapy as a response to mental distress when that distress may be an appropriate response to social disadvantage and inequality (Masson 1988; Furedi 2004; Smail 2005; Moloney 2013).

Case study

Magdalena is approaching the end of her mental health nursing programme and, having enjoyed her time at university, is already considering furthering her studies. In particular, she would like to develop her counselling skills and is thinking about undertaking additional training in order to develop further her ability to incorporate counselling and psychotherapeutic techniques into her practice. However, she has been struck by the wide range of available psychological therapies and is confused about which to pursue and which might be beneficial for those who use mental health services. Although she has only carried out the briefest of internet searches, she has already discovered a wide variety of psychological therapies that are used to respond to mental distress, including cognitive behavioural therapy, dialectical behavioural therapy, existential therapy, solution-focused therapy, interpersonal therapy, mindfulness-based cognitive therapy, mentalisation-based therapy, acceptance and commitment therapy, behavioural family therapy and eye movement desensitisation and reprocessing therapy.

While extensive critical debate surrounds psychological interventions from a multiplicity of perspectives, a key issue that will impact upon the incorporation of counselling and psychotherapeutic skills into your mental health practice concerns the wide variety of available psychological interventions. It has been suggested that there are over 400 different forms of psychological therapies in existence and, like Magdalena in the case study above, you may be feeling overwhelmed by that wide variety as well as being confused about which would be appropriate to seek to incorporate into your mental health practice. However, while the research evidence for the effectiveness of psychological interventions generally, and for the effectiveness of one intervention over another in particular, is both complex and contested, it has repeatedly been asserted that, when different therapeutic approaches are compared with each other, there appears to be minimal difference between them in terms of their effectiveness (Luborsky *et al.* 2002; Cooper 2008; Kelly & Moloney 2013).

Rather than the influence of any specific psychotherapeutic techniques – such as the identification of negative thoughts in cognitive behavioural therapy or interpretations that connect past and present relationships in psychodynamic therapy – 'non-specific factors' are understood to have an equal, if not greater, impact on the clinical effectiveness and outcome of psychological interventions. While a variety of non-specific factors have been identified – such as social support, self-change and fortuitous events – it has been suggested that the most influential non-specific factor on therapeutic effectiveness is the quality of the therapeutic relationship and, in particular, the presence of warmth, empathy, understanding and the instillation of hope (Norcross 2011; Cahill *et al.* 2013; Wampold & Imel 2015). In your daily mental health practice the particular counselling skills and psychotherapeutic techniques that you employ will be inextricably bound to the manner in which you relate to those who use mental health services. However, such critical evaluations of the effectiveness of one psychological intervention over another suggest the importance of giving at least equal consideration to your ability to develop therapeutic relationships and supportive alliances with those who use mental health services as you do to the development and employment of counselling skills and psychotherapeutic techniques.

Activity 6.2   *Evidence-based practice and research*

The National Institute for Health and Care Excellence (NICE) is a non-departmental public body that aims to provide information, advice and standards to improve and maximise the use of evidence across all areas of health and social care. In doing so, it provides national guidelines on how to treat and manage a range of mental health difficulties, including guidance on which psychological therapies are recommended for particular forms of mental distress.

For this activity, go to the NICE website (**www.nice.org.uk**) and, in particular, access the guidelines for the treatment of schizophrenia in adults, entitled 'Psychosis and schizophrenia in adults: treatment and management (CG178)'.

- Which psychological interventions does NICE recommend in the treatment and management of psychosis and schizophrenia?

An outline answer is provided at the end of the chapter.

Service user involvement

The collective action of people who use mental health services in the provision and the development of those services has, over the past 30 years, emerged as one of the most significant features of contemporary mental health care. A commitment to the involvement of service user groups in mental health services is reflected in the principles and policies that guide contemporary mental health practice and those who have received, or who continue to receive, mental health care are increasingly engaged in a wide range of mental health service activities. In particular, service user groups are often consulted about their experiences of mental health care by those who provide mental health services, and such consultancy work not only involves the monitoring and evaluation of existing services, but also contributes to the development of new services; increasingly acknowledged as being 'experts by experience', those who use mental health services are also involved in the recruitment and training of mental health professionals and, among others things, work to promote alternative understandings of mental distress and alternative ways to respond to that distress. In addition, service user groups are engaged in conducting research pertinent to all aspects of contemporary mental health care, and this not only takes the form of contributions to research that is conducted by mental health professionals but, increasingly, there is a focus on the development of service-user-led research (Beresford 2010; Weinstein 2010). Indeed, it has been suggested that it is no longer feasible for any significant discussions about the provision, evaluation and development of mental health services to occur without ensuring the involvement of mental health service user groups; those who use mental health services *are now a presence in aspects of mental health services in which their presence would have been inconceivable a quarter of a century ago; this is an indication of the change in climate that has occurred* (Campbell 2013, p. 140).

Concept summary: The service user/survivor movement

Although the collective action of people who use mental health services has been understood as a new type of social movement, it is important to recognise the differences and diversity that characterise that movement. It has been estimated that there are perhaps more than 600 service user/survivor groups throughout the UK and they are notable both for the diversity of their activities and the variety of assumptions, values and beliefs that inspire those activities (Campbell 2013). Indeed, while the terms 'service user' and 'service survivor' are often linked together, they clearly reflect differing attitudes towards mental health services and differences in the experiences of those people who have used, or who continue to use, those services. Despite such differences, however, a range of common positions, beliefs and activities have been identified that can be understood as broadly characterising the service user/survivor movement. These include:

- a commitment to tackle the stigma, discrimination and exclusion associated with mental distress and a determination to increase the opportunities for greater social inclusion of those with mental health difficulties;
- a suspicion of the dominance of the biomedical approach to understanding mental distress and the associated reliance on physical interventions such as psychiatric medication and ECT;
- an insistence on the right of people who experience mental distress to reclaim and redefine that experience in their own terms and, characteristically, to do so using non-medicalised language;
- a demand for the experiences and expertise of those who use mental health services to be recognised along with the value of service-user-led interventions such as peer support, mentoring and befriending;
- an opposition to the extension of compulsory powers to detain and treat people who experience mental distress and an assertion of the negative impact of custodial practices such as seclusion and restraint.

Despite the increased involvement of service user groups in the provision, evaluation and development of contemporary mental health services, there are continuing critical considerations about the nature of that involvement and the extent to which it can be understood, as it is often presented, as empowering those who use mental health services (Stickley 2006; Stringer *et al.* 2008; Roberts 2010). While it has been suggested that the collective action of service user groups has resulted in a number of significant achievements in mental health care – such as the establishment of independent mental health advocacy – questions remain about the extent to which service user involvement in mental health services is meaningful or simply tokenistic. In particular, a number of barriers have been identified that are said to restrict meaningful service user involvement at the highest levels of the decision-making process, barriers that not only limit the co-production of mental health services but also actively prevent service user groups from taking a lead in the planning, delivery and evaluation of those services. For example, it has been argued that the opinions, experiences and knowledge of mental health professionals is often given greater credibility in the decision-making process than the opinions, experience and knowledge of those who use mental health services; it has also been suggested that there is a lack of genuine commitment to listen actively to, and change as a consequence of, the opinions and experiences expressed by service user groups and, in particular, a reluctance to consider alternative, non-biomedical understandings of mental distress; in addition, the over-reliance on jargon, a lack of appropriate and readily available information, inflexible and bureaucratic organisational systems and insufficient resources have all been identified as restricting the meaningful involvement of people who use mental health services in the provision, evaluation and development of those services (Hitchen *et al.* 2011; Beresford 2013; NSUN 2015a).

Activity 6.3   *Reflection*

One of the principal objectives of service user group involvement in mental health services has been to maximise the participation of individual mental health service users in all aspects of their care and treatment. However, while there is an expectation that mental health professionals will recognise the expertise, and promote the self-determination, of those who use mental health services, it has been suggested that the meaningful involvement of individual service users in their own care and treatment remains limited (McLean *et al.* 2012; Campbell 2013).

For this activity, critically consider your clinical placement experiences and attempt to identify three instances in which those who use mental health services were meaningfully involved in decisions about their care and treatment.

As this activity is based on your own reflections, there is no outline answer at the end of the chapter.

Recovery

While it has been suggested that the meaningful involvement of mental health service users in their care remains limited, it is important to recognise that – unlike many notions that shape how mental distress is understood and responded to in contemporary mental health care – ideas about recovery can be understood as originating from, and being profoundly influenced by, the personal accounts of people who have had direct experience of mental distress and who have used mental health services (Chamberlin 1977; Deegan 1988; Coleman 1999). Over recent years, the notion of recovery has increasingly gained attention from, and been adopted by, academics, researchers and mental health professionals, such that there is now an explicit emphasis on practising in a recovery-focused way in the literature, research and policy that guide contemporary mental health care (Anthony 1993; Repper & Perkins 2003; DH 2011a). However, despite the reorientation of mental health services towards recovery-focused principles and practice, it is important to recognise that recovery continues to be a complex, multidimensional and contested concept. For example, there exist critical debates about the extent to which the notion of recovery is applicable to the various forms of mental distress that people experience and whether a recovery-focused approach can realistically be adopted in all of the settings in which contemporary mental health care occurs; there are also critical questions about what personal, organisational and social conditions are necessary to facilitate recovery, as well as competing suggestions about how to monitor, measure and determine an individual's recovery progress. In addition, there are provocative analyses about the role that mental health services should have in facilitating recovery and whether, in being adopted by the mental health professions, recovery has been incorporated into, and distorted by, what are seen as the traditionally paternalistic practices of psychiatry (Roberts 2008; Pilgrim & McCranie 2013; Repper & Perkins 2014).

Case study

Seamus is a 32-year-old man who has a history of depression, self-harm and alcohol use problems and has had a series of mental health hospital admissions over the past three years. Several days ago he was admitted to hospital under section 3 of the Mental Health Act 1983 after his mood appeared to deteriorate rapidly and he made an attempt to commit suicide. On admission he was assessed as being 'a significant suicide risk' and was placed on one-to-one observations. However, he became increasingly dissatisfied with this intervention and, when informed by staff that this level of observation was temporary but, at present, necessary, he began to express a desire to return home. Earlier this afternoon, the staff on the ward reported that Seamus had been displaying aggressive behaviour towards other people and, following an argument with an agency staff member, had attempted to leave the ward. In order to prevent him from doing so he was restrained by four members of staff and subsequently placed in a seclusion room.

While there exist a number of critical debates surrounding the notion of recovery, one of the most enduring concerns the extent to which a recovery-orientated approach can be reconciled with the range of functions that are expected of contemporary mental health services. In particular, a fundamental critical question concerns the extent to which the recovery-focused reorientation of mental health services can be accommodated with the need to assess and manage the risks effectively that those who experience mental distress can potentially pose to themselves and to others. You may already be aware that there exists mental health legislation that permits an individual's autonomy and self-determination to be constrained, as in the above case study, if doing so is judged to be in the best interests of that individual's health, safety or for the protection of others. However, it has been suggested that such legal powers, and the requirement for mental health services to manage risk more generally, are seemingly incompatible with a recovery-orientated approach: while the assumptions, values and beliefs that inform recovery are concerned with fostering hope, facilitating involvement and maximising personal control, the employment of mental health legislation and the management of risk are said to be associated with imposing restrictions, ensuring containment and asserting staff control (Pilgrim & McCranie 2013; Repper & Perkins 2014). However, it has been argued that the employment of mental health legislation, and the effective management of risk more generally, need not necessarily be understood as being incompatible with a recovery-focused approach; in particular, it has been suggested that it is possible to manage crisis and risk in a way that strives to maximise involvement, collaboration and independence such that a person is increasingly able to share, and then take responsibility for, any decisions made in order to move towards re-establishing control over his or her own life (Morgan 2013; Boardman & Roberts 2014).

Activity 6.4	*Reflection*

The extent to which a recovery-focused approach can be reconciled with the range of responsibilities that contemporary mental health services are expected to meet is a complex and challenging one which you should consider as you progress through your mental health nursing programme. However, as a mental health nursing student it will be productive to begin to reflect critically upon the extent to which you are practising in a way that can be meaningfully referred to as recovery-focused in the variety of settings in which you will work.

In order to help mental health professionals assess the extent to which their practice is recovery-focused, a series of reflective questions have been proposed (Shepherd *et al.* 2008; Roberts & Boardman 2014). Consider your clinical experiences so far, and your interactions with those who use mental health services in particular, and use these questions to reflect critically upon the extent to which your practice has been, or is developing towards becoming, recovery-focused. In particular, when you work with those who use mental health services:

- Do you actively listen to assist the person to make sense of his or her mental health problems?
- Do you help the person identify and prioritise his or her personal goals for recovery and not the goals that you believe s/he ought to pursue?
- Do you demonstrate a belief in the person's existing strengths and resources in relation to the pursuit of these goals?
- Do you identify examples from your own lived experience, or the experiences of other mental health service users, which inspire and validate their hopes?
- Do you pay particular attention to the importance of goals which take the person out of the 'sick role' and enable him or her to contribute actively to the lives of others?

continued . . .

- Do you identify non-mental health resources – such as friends, family and wider agencies – that may be relevant to the achievement of these goals?
- Do you encourage self-management of mental distress by providing information, reinforcing existing coping strategies and facilitating the development of new skills?
- Do you discuss what the person wants in terms of therapeutic interventions, including physical and psychological interventions, and do you respect the individual's wishes wherever possible?
- Do you behave at all times so as to convey an attitude of respect for the person and a desire for an equal working partnership?
- Do you accept that the future is uncertain and that setbacks will happen, while facilitating hope, maintaining positive expectations and continuing to express support for the possibility of the person achieving his or her self-defined goals?

As this activity is based on your own reflections, there is no outline answer at the end of the chapter.

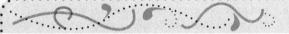

Chapter summary

This chapter has highlighted and discussed a variety of critical considerations surrounding the interventions used in contemporary mental health care and the involvement of those people who use mental health services in that care. In particular, those considerations have been situated within the context of four broad areas of contemporary mental health practice: first, with regard to the intervention that those who use mental health services are most likely to receive, a number of critical issues surrounding psychiatric medication have been highlighted and, in particular, critical questions that are concerned with how psychiatric drugs work; second, despite psychological treatments being the interventions that those who use mental health services commonly express a general preference for, this chapter has introduced various provocative critical considerations surrounding their function, employment and effectiveness; third, a number of critical questions have been raised about the increased involvement of those people who use mental health services in all aspects of those services and, in particular, critical concerns about the extent to which that involvement can be understood as meaningful or simply tokenistic; and finally, this chapter has highlighted various critical issues surrounding the notion of recovery and the extent to which a recovery-focused approach can be reconciled with the range of responsibilities that contemporary mental health services are expected to meet. In presenting this range of critical issues about psychiatric medication, psychological interventions, service user involvement and the notion of recovery, this chapter has encouraged you to begin to think critically about their implications for your own mental health nursing practice in order to enable you to become an informed, proactive and increasingly critically reflective mental health practitioner.

Activities: brief outline answers

Activity 6.1 Critical thinking

The manner in which you understand how psychiatric drugs work will potentially have far-reaching implications for your mental health nursing practice and, in particular, the manner in which you assist those who use mental health services to make informed choices about psychiatric medication. Insofar as the disease-centred model presents psychiatric drugs as targeting specific underlying biological dysfunctions, it has been suggested that mental health professionals might be led to assume that any adverse effects of psychiatric drugs should be understood by mental health service users as a tolerable by-product of what is ultimately a beneficial and therapeutic physical intervention (Moncrieff *et al.* 2013). In contrast, understood as psychoactive substances that act on the central nervous system to produce a range of altered mental and physical states, the drug-centred model can lead mental health professionals to give equal consideration to all of the effects that a given psychiatric drug may produce and to discuss those effects with those who use mental health services. Rather than minimising the potentially adverse effects of psychiatric medication – and the active involvement of mental health service users in discussions about the effects of, and alternatives to, that medication – the drug-centred model enables those who use mental health services to consider which drug-induced mental and physical states they might find beneficial and which states they might not. In doing so, it has been suggested that *the drug-centred model provides a rationale for periodic rather than continuous drug use, to cope with exacerbations of symptoms or to palliate stressful environmental events and avoid the harm associated with long term use* (Moncrieff & Cohen 2009, p. 2).

Activity 6.2 Evidence-based practice and research

In accessing the NICE guidelines for the treatment and management of psychosis and schizophrenia, you will have noticed that different psychological interventions are recommended depending on whether those interventions are concerned with *preventing psychosis*, with *first-episode psychosis*, with *subsequent acute episodes of psychosis or schizophrenia and referral in psychosis* or with *promoting recovery and possible future care*. However, you should have identified that NICE advises offering cognitive behavioural therapy to all people deemed to be experiencing an episode of psychosis or diagnosed with schizophrenia; NICE also recommends offering family intervention to all families of people deemed to be experiencing an episode of psychosis or diagnosed with schizophrenia and who live with, or who are in close contact with, the mental health service user; finally, NICE recommends considering the provision of arts therapies to all people deemed to be experiencing an episode of psychosis or diagnosed with schizophrenia, particularly for the alleviation of the so-called 'negative symptoms'.

Further reading

Beresford P (2010) *A Straight Talking Introduction to Being a Mental Health Service User.* Ross-on-Wye: PCCS Books.

This book provides a comprehensive introduction to the mental health service user/survivor movement which includes, among other things, a discussion of how to move towards meaningful service user involvement in mental health services.

Moncrieff J (2008) *The Myth of the Chemical Cure: A critique of psychiatric drug treatment.* Basingstoke: Palgrave Macmillan.

Here you will find a sustained critical account of the disease-centred and the drug-centred explanations of how psychiatric medication works, along with a discussion about the implications of the drug-centred model for those who use, and those who work within, mental health services.

Pilgrim D (2009) *A Straight Talking Introduction to Psychological Treatments for Mental Health Problems.* Ross-on-Wye: PCCS Books.

This book provides a comprehensive introduction to a variety of critical issues surrounding the function, the employment and the effectiveness of psychological interventions as a response to mental distress.

Pilgrim D & McCranie A (2013) *Recovery and Mental Health: A critical sociological account.* Basingstoke: Palgrave Macmillan.

A stimulating examination of the concept of recovery from a critical sociological perspective which includes a discussion of the apparent conflict between mental health legislation and recovery-focused practice.

Useful websites

www.bacp.co.uk

This is the website for the British Association for Counselling and Psychotherapy (BACP), which is the largest professional body representing counselling and psychotherapy in the UK, and which provides a wide range of information about a variety of issues pertinent to counselling and psychotherapy.

www.nsun.org.uk

Here you will find the website for the National Survivor User Network. This is an independent, service-user-led charity that provides advice, support and information to promote active and meaningful mental health service user/survivor involvement.

Chapter 7
Academic standards

NMC Standards for Pre-registration Nursing Education

This chapter will address the following competencies:

Domain 1: Professional values

7   All nurses must be responsible and accountable for keeping their knowledge and skills up to date through continuing professional development. They must aim to improve their performance and enhance the safety and quality of care through evaluation, supervision and appraisal.

Domain 2: Communication and interpersonal skills

3   All nurses must use the full range of communication methods, including verbal, non-verbal and written, to acquire, interpret and record their knowledge and understanding of people's needs. They must be aware of their own values and beliefs and the impact this may have on their communication with others. They must take account of the many different ways in which people communicate and how these may be influenced by ill health, disability and other factors, and be able to recognise and respond effectively when a person finds it hard to communicate.

Chapter aims

By the end of this chapter you will be able to:

- identify the range of academic standards that are used to assess the quality of critical thinking and critical reflection;
- understand the academic standards that are commonly used to assess the content of critical thinking and critical reflection;
- understand the academic standards that are commonly used to assess the form of critical thinking and reflection.

Introduction

Case study

Riya is midway through her mental health nursing programme and, while she is doing well on her clinical practice placements, she is becoming increasingly concerned about the grades that she has been

continued . . .

receiving for her university assignments. Although her grades were low at the beginning of the course, they began to improve towards the end of the first year; however, her grades at the beginning of the second year became progressively worse and, to her disappointment, she has just found out that she has failed her most recent assignment. Although she reads the feedback on her work carefully, she has found that she receives comments from her tutors that she is unsure how to address, such as 'your work is a little superficial at times', 'more clarity of expression required' and 'avoid making unsubstantiated claims'. As a consequence she is becoming increasingly confused about why the grades that she receives are so inconsistent and she is keen to understand what she needs to do not only to ensure that her grades are good but, more importantly, that they are consistently good.

Just as there are standards against which your clinical work and conduct as a mental health nursing student can be assessed, so too are there standards against which your academic work generally, and your critical thinking and reflective capabilities in particular, can be assessed. In order to monitor, measure and develop these critical capabilities consistently for your academic work then it will be necessary to gain an understanding of, and strive to work in accordance with, those academic standards. Indeed, doing so will not only be beneficial for your university assignments – and, as Riya is keen to discover in the above case study, will enable you to understand how to ensure that your academic work is consistently good – but will also help you to monitor, measure and develop your critical thinking and reflective capabilities for your mental health practice. However, a variety of academic standards have been proposed and these are subject to critical discussion, debate and interpretation (Paul & Elder 2014); indeed, it is likely that your university has produced its own guidance on the standards against which your academic work will be assessed and you should access, read and consider these carefully. Despite this diversity, it is possible to recognise a number of common academic standards and, in doing so, it is productive to note a general distinction between those that are concerned with the content of your academic work, with what it is that you say, and those that are concerned with the form of your academic work, with how it is that you express what you have to say. In practice, both the content and the form of your academic work will be inextricably linked and, in order to develop your ability to produce consistently high-quality university assignments, it will be necessary to develop both an understanding of the academic standards that relate to the content of your work and those that relate to the form by which you express that content.

The purpose of this chapter is to introduce you to the standards against which your academic work generally, and your critical thinking and reflective capabilities in particular, can be assessed. However, while a variety of academic standards exist, this chapter will begin by examining three standards that are commonly employed to assess the content of academic work; in particular, we shall examine the manner in which the 'relevance' of your work can be assessed, the degree to which you adequately respond to what is asked of you in your academic assignments; we shall then examine the manner in which academic work is often assessed for the 'depth' of critical thinking and reflection that it displays; in addition, we shall discuss the manner in which that work is commonly assessed for the 'breadth' of thought and understanding that it demonstrates. However, after examining the academic standards that are concerned with the content of your academic work, this chapter will then discuss the standards by which the form of that work can be assessed. Again, while a variety of such standards have been proposed, this chapter will examine three standards that are commonly employed to assess the form of academic work; in particular, we shall discuss the manner in which the style of your work is assessed, with how it is that you express what you have to say; we shall then examine the manner in which your ability to demonstrate competence with referencing your work is assessed; finally, we shall discuss the manner in which your ability to display competence with grammar, punctuation and spelling throughout your university assignments is assessed. Acquiring a comprehensive understanding of these academic standards, and how to monitor, measure and develop your work in accordance with them, will take time, practice and patience; however, throughout this chapter you will be encouraged to think about, and strive to work in accordance with, these standards in order to begin to develop your ability to produce consistently high-quality academic assignments for your mental health nursing programme.

Relevance

Case study

Caroline and Tony, two mental health nursing students, are discussing an essay question that they have recently been set in which they are required, in no more than 2,000 words, to 'Provide a detailed account of the stress-vulnerability model in the context of schizophrenia and discuss how it influences choices about which therapeutic interventions to provide'. Although she remembers being taught about the stress-vulnerability model, Caroline states that she is finding the essay difficult because she is unsure how that model influences decisions about which interventions to provide. However, Tony says that he is finding the essay relatively straightforward and has enjoyed writing it because it has enabled him to research into, and make interesting connections between, the work of R.D. Laing, Marius Romme and Mary Boyle. In particular, he tells Caroline that he has used that work to suggest that, in contrast to the biomedical model of mental distress, the experiences of those with a diagnosis of schizophrenia may be understood as intelligible if placed within the context of their individual life history and particular present circumstances.

One of the most fundamental academic standards against which your work will be assessed concerns the degree to which the content of that work, what it is that you have to say, is relevant to what is being asked of you. You may be confident, like Tony in the above case study, that you have produced an informed, insightful and innovative piece of academic work, but if it does not adequately address the question that has been asked of you then it is unlikely to meet the academic requirement of being relevant. Before you begin to address any assignment that you are set over the duration of your mental health nursing programme, it is therefore important to spend a sufficient amount of time considering what is required of you and this will almost certainly involve attempting to clarify the meaning of the assignment question. Doing so will enable you to begin to think about the content of your work in a structured, systematic and coherent manner that will help you determine what material to include in your assignments and, ultimately, reduce the possibility of including material that is irrelevant. However, even if you have clarified what is required of you in an academic assignment, as you begin to consider what material to include in your work you may discover that you are able to identify various forms of information, knowledge and research that could be considered relevant to the question that you have been set. While there may be a wide range of material that could be considered relevant to what has been asked of you and that you could potentially include in your work, it is important to recognise that not all of that material may be equally relevant. Indeed, part of the challenge in ensuring that the content of your work is relevant involves being able to determine what is the most relevant material with respect to what is being asked of you, to be able to determine from the wide range of potentially relevant material what it is necessary to include in your assignment and what material can be omitted.

Activity 7.1   *Decision making*

In the above case study it may be that Tony is able to argue that what he is intending to include in his essay is relevant to the assignment question that has been set. However, given that he is required to respond to that question in no more than 2,000 words, the key issue is whether it is the most relevant material to include in order to address the question that has been asked.

For this activity, carefully consider the assignment question in which Caroline and Tony have been asked to 'Provide a detailed account of the stress-vulnerability model in the context of schizophrenia and discuss how it influences choices about which therapeutic interventions to provide'. In particular, briefly outline what you think it would be necessary to include in the essay in order to ensure that it satisfactorily addresses the question that has been asked.

An outline answer is provided at the end of the chapter.

Depth

Case study

Lilia has just received the feedback for a second-year assignment on her mental health nursing programme in which she was asked to reflect critically upon therapeutic communication in the context of one of her clinical practice placements. Although she has passed the assignment, the tutor has identified that she has made a number of grammatical, punctuation and referencing errors, and has also suggested that her work is 'a little superficial at times' and 'lacking in depth'. Lilia is surprised by these comments because she tried particularly hard to include everything in her essay that she learned about therapeutic communication during the module and, more generally, what she has learned over the duration of her mental health nursing course so far. For example, she provided an overview of

continued . . .

> non-verbal communication and linked it to a description of Egan's (2014) SOLER model, which
> suggests the need to face clients squarely, adopt an open posture, lean towards the other, main-
> tain appropriate eye contact and, finally, to try to relax throughout the interaction. In addition,
> she included a list of verbal techniques such as summarising, paraphrasing and the use of open and
> closed questions; also, she set both verbal and non-verbal communication within the context of a
> description of the **core conditions** necessary to establish therapeutic relationships: empathy, genuine-
> ness and unconditional positive regard.

Over the duration of your mental health nursing programme you will be introduced to
various forms of information, knowledge and research and, at least in the academic setting,
you will be expected to display your understanding of this material in your university assignments. However, it is important to recognise that if, like Lilia in the case study above, you
display such understanding by consistently listing, describing or providing an overview of
what you have learned, then your work is likely to be considered as superficial and lacking
in depth. As you progress through your mental health nursing programme it will not be
sufficient simply to reproduce what you have been taught; rather, you will also be expected
to 'get beneath the surface' of the material to which you have been introduced. In particular, this means that you will be required to think critically about, and reflect critically upon,
that material in order to identify, and actively engage with, the complexities that are often
associated with what you have been taught. As we have suggested, contemporary mental
health care is a complex, challenging and often contested field of health care, and your
academic assignments provide you with an opportunity to display your ability to identify,
and critically engage with, the varied complexities, multiple perspectives and challenging
issues that are associated with many aspects of the theory and practice of that field of health
care. While it can be tempting to simplify, disregard or even deny this complexity, in order
to begin to display a depth of thought about the field of health care into which you are
entering then it will be important to develop a sense of, and to feel confident engaging
with, this complexity. Indeed, one of the most productive ways in which you can begin to
develop a sense of the complexities that are associated with the theory and the practice of
contemporary mental health care – and, by doing so, introduce a depth of thought and
understanding into your academic work – is to be willing to question the material to which
you are being introduced and, in particular, to question that which is often accepted as
being self-evident.

Activity 7.2   *Critical thinking*

Like Lilia in the above case study, you may already have been introduced to what are often
considered to be the core conditions necessary to establish therapeutic relationships in
mental health nursing: empathy, genuineness and unconditional positive regard. Indeed,
they are considered so fundamental that their meaning, value and applicability are commonly accepted as being self-evident and, as a consequence, they are often dealt with in a

continued . . .

superficial, cursory and uncritical manner. However, for this activity, attempt to 'get beneath the surface' of one of those core conditions by critically considering the following definition of unconditional positive regard provided by Carl Rogers (2004, p. 62):

> *It means that the therapist cares for the client, in a non-possessive way. It means that he prizes the client in a total rather than a conditional way. By this I mean that he does not simply accept the client when he is behaving in certain ways, and disapproves of him when he behaves in other ways. It means an outgoing positive feeling without reservations, without evaluations.*

- Given this definition, what would you have to do, in practical terms, to be considered as displaying unconditional positive regard?
- How achievable do you think it is to maintain an *outgoing positive feeling without reservations, without evaluations?*
- Is it possible to disapprove of some behaviours and still 'prize' a person *in a total rather than a conditional way?*

As this activity is based on your own critical thinking, there is no outline answer at the end of the chapter.

Breadth

Case study

*Daniel is approaching the end of his mental health nursing programme and, earlier today, finished his final university examination. Although he is relieved to have no more examinations, he is beginning to reflect upon one of the questions and, in particular, that which asked him to 'Identify and critically discuss the social determinants of mental health'. In answering this question, Daniel focused on the link between labour-market position and mental health and, with reference to contemporary research, discussed the suggestion that, while unemployment is associated with mental distress, it is low-paid, insecure employment that has the largest detrimental effect on a person's mental health. However, after discussing this question with his colleagues, and the variety of other **social determinants** that they have identified, Daniel is beginning to think that he may not have done as well as he had initially thought. In particular, he thinks that he may have focused too narrowly on the link between labour-market position and mental health and perhaps should have broadened out his discussion to include the variety of other social determinants of mental health.*

Although your academic work will commonly be assessed for the depth of critical thought that it displays, as well as the degree to which you adequately respond to what is being asked of you in your university assignments, it will also be assessed for the breadth of thought and understanding that it demonstrates. However, demonstrating a breadth of thought and understanding in your work can be a particular challenge, not least because what it means to do so can be understood in a variety of interrelated ways. For example, like Daniel's answer to the examination question in the above case study, it may be that the focus of your work is too 'narrow' insofar as it does not sufficiently discuss other factors, issues or topics that may be relevant to what is being asked of you; similarly, it may be that you have not included, for example, prominent thinkers, key ideas or established pieces of research in your work and have therefore failed to demonstrate that you have adequately reviewed, and sufficiently 'read around', the topic under consideration; in addition, it may be that you have not acknowledged that there are multiple perspectives on a particular issue or, while acknowledging other perspectives, they have been misrepresented or disregarded without reasoned justification.

There may therefore be a variety of reasons why a piece of academic work has been judged to have failed to demonstrate sufficient breadth of thought and understanding and you should develop a sensitivity for, and seek to address, the potential presence of the foregoing failings in your own work. However, as was discussed in Chapter 3, one of the most significant obstacles to critical thinking and reflection, and which can substantially restrict your ability to demonstrate a breadth of thought and understanding in your university assignments, is egocentrism or the tendency to adhere to a single perspective without giving due consideration to alternative perspectives. Seeking to address the potential presence of egocentrism in your academic work, and thereby ensuring that it displays a breadth of thought and understanding, does not mean that you cannot develop, maintain and defend your own perspective and position with respect to the area or issue of mental health care under investigation; rather, it entails acknowledging that your perspective is situated within a broader context of critical thought, research and discussion as well as demonstrating a willingness to represent accurately, consider seriously and engage critically with the variety of perspectives which characterise that context.

Activity 7.3   *Decision making*

Re-read the above case study and consider the examination question in which Daniel was asked to 'Identify and critically discuss the social determinants of mental health'. In particular, identify what other social determinants, apart from labour-market position, you could have included in an answer to this question in order to demonstrate a breadth of thought and understanding.

An outline answer is provided at the end of the chapter.

Style

In order to begin to develop your ability to produce consistently high-quality academic work on your mental health nursing programme that is characterised by critical thinking and reflection, it is necessary to become aware of, and work in accordance with, the standards against which the content of that work is commonly assessed. However, it is important to recognise that the content of your work, what it is that you have to say, will be inextricably linked to the form of your work, with how it is that you express what you have to say. It is therefore also necessary to become aware of, and work in accordance with, the standards against which the form of your work will be assessed, and one of the most important of these standards is concerned with the style of writing that you adopt for your university assignments. As you progress through your mental health nursing programme, you will become increasingly aware that there is a particular style of writing that is considered appropriate for university assignments, a style of writing that is characterised by a variety of rules, conventions and expectations. Indeed, your university is likely to possess its own guidelines on 'academic style' and you should access, read and consider these carefully in order to begin to clarify what style of writing and expression is expected of you in your academic work.

Concept summary: Academic style

Providing a comprehensive definition of what constitutes an academic style of writing can be a particular challenge because it refers to writing that is conducted across a variety of academic disciplines, in various contexts and is adopted, adapted and occasionally even resisted in order to serve a variety of intellectual purposes. However, an academic style of writing can be understood as possessing a number of common characteristics and it has been suggested that there are a number of things that you should avoid doing in order to begin to develop a style of writing that can be considered appropriate for your university assignments (Osmond 2013; Price & Harrington 2013). For example, you should avoid:

- contractions, or shortened versions of words (such as 'don't', 'they'll' and 'it's'); instead, always use the full form (such as 'do not', 'they will' and 'it is');
- complicated, elaborate words or jargon; of course, in mental health nursing it may be necessary to use technical, clinical words but you should make sure that you demonstrate a clear understanding of those words;
- clichés or phrases and expressions that have been used so often that they have lost their effectiveness, such as 'at the end of the day', 'the fact of the matter' and 'in the final analysis';
- slang, colloquialisms or informal words and phrases that are commonly used in everyday spoken language, such as 'kids', 'a load of issues' or 'a pretty good point';
- emotive language, or words and phrases that are used to argue, influence and persuade by appealing to the emotions, such as 'a cowardly, shameful way to behave' or 'a vicious, barbaric intervention';
- the 'first person', such as 'I', 'we', 'my', 'us' and 'ours', unless otherwise instructed (such as may occur in a piece of reflective writing). Where possible use the 'third person'; for example: 'It can be argued' instead of 'I think';
- discriminatory, exclusionary or potentially offensive language, including words and phrases that perpetuate stereotypes on the basis of age, disability, ethnicity, gender, mental health, nationality, sexuality, socio-economic status and spirituality.

Activity 7.4   *Team working*

An important aspect of developing a competent academic writing style for your university assignments, and an important aspect of developing your critical mental health nursing practice more generally, is to gain a sensitivity to the use of language in contemporary mental health care. Rather than simply describing the world in a neutral, value-free manner, the language that we use can be understood as being informed by a variety of assumptions, values and beliefs and as being profoundly influential in producing, maintaining and changing how we understand and respond to the world (Bourdieu 1992; Foucault 2005; Fairclough 2015).

For this activity, consider the use of the following terms used in contemporary mental health care and, with your colleagues, discuss the appropriateness of using them in your university assignments:

- mental illness;
- mental health difficulty;
- mental distress;
- madness.

An outline answer is provided at the end of the chapter.

The rules, conventions and expectations that are characteristic of the writing style that is considered appropriate for your university assignments can take time to incorporate into your academic work. Indeed, it is sometimes thought that this can be made more challenging when attempting to demonstrate critical thinking and critical reflection in your work because it may require you to explain, engage with and develop what can be potentially complex ideas. However, it is important to recognise that any reader of your academic work expects to be able to understand what it is that you have to say and, to that end, also expects that you will be attempting to communicate as effectively as possible. Indeed, it has been suggested that you should not be misled by the word 'style' into thinking that, because you are studying at university level, you are required to use elaborate, convoluted sentences and obscure, complex words (Peck & Coyle 2012). Rather, the overarching aim for your university assignments should be to strive continually to express your ideas – and especially those that others may find complex and challenging – in a simple, concise and clear manner by adopting and developing an academic style of writing that is focused on facilitating understanding.

References

Case study

Elizabeth, a first-year mental health nursing student, is currently in a tutorial in which the lecturer, Dr Miller, is discussing the requirements for this semester's module assignment. Elizabeth remembers that on her last assignment she received feedback which stated that she had made 'a number of unsubstantiated claims' and was advised to support the claims that she was making with 'argument, research and evidence'.

---

continued . . .

> *In particular, it was suggested that there was a notable lack of referencing throughout her work and she was informed to make more use of the available literature. Elizabeth is keen to address the feedback that she receives on her university assignments in order to improve her academic writing and, ultimately, her grades; therefore, when Dr Miller asks if anybody has any questions about the essay that is required for this semester's module, Elizabeth asks how many references she should include in her work this time.*

The use of references – which means providing a record of the sources that you have used to explain points, discuss issues and develop arguments in your work – is an essential feature of high-quality academic writing. Indeed, your university will almost certainly have produced guidelines on the importance of referencing your work, which referencing system you are required to use and how to reference correctly the variety of material that you are likely to include in your assignments. Despite this, an understanding of the purpose, importance and correct method of using references in academic writing can sometimes appear to be lacking in university assignments; indeed, while Elizabeth's question about references in the above case study may be understandable in the context of the feedback that she received on her previous assignment, it perhaps reflects an assumption that references are not integral to academic writing and that the measure of good referencing is determined by the quantity that appear in an assignment. However, it is important that you do begin to understand references as an essential aspect of your academic work that can contribute to the establishment and maintenance of your reputation as an honest, considerate and conscientious student of mental health nursing. In order to understand how, it is necessary to recognise that your academic work will be situated within a broader context of critical thought, research and discussion and, in your university assignments, you will invariably explain points, discuss issues and develop arguments by drawing upon the ideas, opinions and research of others. In this context, referencing serves a variety of functions: it is, for example, a form of professional courtesy and honesty in which you indicate when you have used someone else's ideas, arguments and even words (indeed, not to indicate when you have done so constitutes **plagiarism**, which is a serious academic offence that can have far-reaching consequences); the use of references also signals that you have researched the topic under discussion, considered the perspectives of others and that your own work is informed by theory, research and evidence. In addition, the use of references provides your readers with valuable information, indicating where they may go to investigate further the work that you have highlighted and which can thereby assist in the learning, development and research of others (Gimenez 2011; Taylor 2013).

Activity 7.5   *Evidence-based practice and research*

Making appropriate reference to prominent thinkers, significant theories and established pieces of research in your work can contribute to the sense that it is characterised by a breadth of thought and understanding. You can often discover these key references by, for example, a brief internet search or by looking at the reference list in your module

continued . . .

guides, and the inclusion and informed use of them in your work can signal to your reader that you are aware of both the historical and current intellectual context in which you are working.

As you may be aware, critical thinking and reflection have been, and continue to be, a characteristic feature of mental health care; indeed, the so-called 'anti-psychiatry' movement and, most recently, the 'critical psychiatry' movement attest to this enduring presence of critical thought and reflection in mental health care. For this activity, iden-tify two prominent thinkers who are often closely associated with the anti-psychiatry movement and, for each thinker, provide a reference for one of his or her influential books.

An outline answer is provided at the end of the chapter.

Grammar, punctuation and spelling

While the form of your academic work will commonly be assessed in terms of the style of writing that you adopt for your academic assignments, and the degree to which you compe-tently reference your work, you will also be assessed for your ability to display competence with respect to grammar, punctuation and spelling. Insofar as your overarching aim in your university assignments should be to express your ideas in a simple, concise and clear manner, then the competent use of grammar, punctuation and spelling can be an essential element in helping you achieve this aim. Conversely, while occasional errors are unlikely seriously to impede an understanding of your work, consistently poor grammar, punctuation and spell-ing can interrupt, restrict and even obscure the meaning of what you are trying to express in your university assignments. Therefore, it has been suggested that as a university student you ought to strive to possess, as a minimum, a competent understanding of grammar, punc-tuation and spelling. In particular, you should not only be able to write sentences that are grammatically correct, but you should also understand how those sentences combine to form coherent paragraphs. In addition, while it is desirable to develop competence with the full range of available punctuation marks, in order to write in a clear manner for your university assignments it is necessary, as a minimum, to understand how to use the full stop, the comma and the apostrophe. Finally, it is expected that you will not only spell words correctly but also be able to identify the correct spelling and meaning between words that sound alike, such as 'their' and 'there', 'effect' and 'affect' and 'practise' and 'practice' (Copus 2009; Peck & Coyle 2012). Again, like many of the skills discussed throughout this chapter, your ability to demonstrate competence with grammar, punctuation and spelling can take time, practice and patience to develop; however, your ability to do so will provide you with increased con-trol over your work, enable you to express yourself with a greater degree of clarity and can ultimately contribute to the improvement of your grades on your mental health nursing programme.

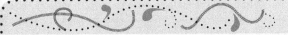

Chapter summary

In this chapter we have highlighted and discussed a number of standards against which your academic work generally, and your critical thinking and reflective capabilities in particular, can be assessed. While a variety of such academic standards exist, we have suggested that it is productive to make a distinction between those that are concerned with the content of your academic work, with what it is that you say, and those that are concerned with the form of your academic work, with how it is that you express what you have to say. In doing so, this chapter has examined three standards that are commonly employed to assess the content of academic work; in particular, it has discussed the manner in which your work is assessed for its relevance, for the depth of critical thinking and reflection that it displays and for the breadth of thought and understanding that it demonstrates. In addition, this chapter has also examined three standards that are commonly employed to assess the form of academic work; in particular, it has discussed the manner in which your work is assessed for the style of writing that you adopt in your academic assignments, the degree to which you display competence with using references in those assignments and, finally, the manner in which you display competence with grammar, punctuation and spelling. Acquiring a comprehensive understanding of these academic standards, and how to monitor, measure and develop your work in accordance with them, ought to be a central concern throughout your university studies; therefore, this chapter has encouraged you to begin to think about, and strive to work in accordance with, these standards in order to ensure that you begin to develop your ability to produce consistently high-quality academic work for your mental health nursing programme.

Activities: brief outline answers

Activity 7.1 Decision making

In deciding what you think it would be necessary to include in the essay that Caroline and Tony have been set you should have identified the need to provide a detailed explanation of the stress-vulnerability model. In doing so, you may have made reference to the work of Zubin and Spring (1977) and also the development of the stress-vulnerability model by contemporary researchers. In particular, you may have identified the need to define and make a distinction between inherited and acquired vulnerabilities and, similarly, the need to define and provide an account of different forms of stress and challenging life events. Importantly, you should have noted the need to include a discussion about the manner in which the stress-vulnerability model suggests that the experience of schizophrenia is to be understood as a consequence of an interaction between a person's specific vulnerabilities and the particular stress to which s/he is subject. In addition, you should have identified the need to discuss how the stress-vulnerability model provides a rationale for specific forms of mental health care interventions. For example, you may have noted how the model's account of inherited, and specifically biological, vulnerability provides a rationale for the use of psychiatric medication. However, you may also have identified the need to include a discussion about how the model's focus on the interaction between acquired vulnerabilities and various forms of stress provides a rationale for the employment of a variety of psychosocial interventions; in particular, you may have noted the manner in which a number of interventions – such as cognitive behavioural therapy, mindfulness-based therapy, family intervention and behavioural activation – can be used by mental health nurses to develop specific strategies to respond, address and even resolve a person's particular vulnerabilities and susceptibility to specific forms of stress (Rayner 2014; Turton 2015).

Activity 7.3 Decision making

In response to the examination question that Daniel was set, there are a number of social determinants, apart from labour-market position, that could have been included in an answer to this question in order to demonstrate a breadth of thought and understanding. For example, you could have made reference to the relationship between mental health and social class, socio-economic status and poverty more generally; you could also have discussed how urbanicity, the quality of housing and the neighbourhoods in which people live affect mental health; in addition, you could have included a discussion about social capital – the degree of participation in, and the value associated with, social networks – and, for example, the distinction between 'bonding', 'bridging' and 'linking' social capital; finally, in discussing the social determinants of mental health you could have highlighted the potentially negative effects of having contact with mental health services, including the socially stigmatising consequences of receiving a psychiatric diagnosis (Lauder *et al.* 2007; Elliot & Masters 2009; Rogers & Pilgrim 2014; WHO 2014).

Activity 7.4 Team working

In considering a number of terms that are employed in contemporary mental health care, and the appropriateness of using those terms in your university assignments, you may have had complex, stimulating and thought-provoking discussions with your colleagues. In particular, those discussions may have been broadly concerned with the manner in which the language that is employed to account for the experiences of those who use mental health services reflects certain assumptions, values and beliefs and, in doing so, is influential in determining how we understand and respond to those experiences. For example, you may have noted that the term mental illness is closely associated with a biological, or what is often referred to as a medical or biomedical, understanding of a person's experience, while mental health difficulty or mental health problem are often used as alternative terms in order to reflect a less biomedical understanding. In addition, you might have discussed the manner in which the term mental distress, and even 'person with direct or lived experience of mental distress', is increasingly favoured as an attempt to emphasise each person's unique lived experience and to recognise the person that exists prior to, and in spite of, any term, label or diagnostic category (Cromby *et al.* 2013b; NSUN 2015b). Finally, in considering the term madness you may have discussed how it has been used to stigmatise, discriminate and exclude those who use mental health services; however, you may also have identified that there have been attempts to reclaim the term by service user organisations such as Mad Pride (Curtis *et al.* 2000). Similarly, while identifying the need to be cautious about using the term madness in your academic assignments because of its past pejorative connotations, you may also have discussed how it is increasingly being used in academic literature that seeks to distance itself from the theoretical assumptions and clinical interventions associated with the discipline of psychiatry (e.g. LeFrançois *et al.* 2013).

Activity 7.5 Evidence-based practice and research

In conducting your own research into the anti-psychiatry movement you may have discovered a number of prominent thinkers, and a variety of influential books, that are often closely associated with that movement. While not an exhaustive list, you may have identified, for example, R.D. Laing's (1960) *The Divided Self*, Thomas Szasz's (1961) *The Myth of Mental Illness*, Michel Foucault's (2001) *Madness and Civilization* and Erving Goffman's (1961) *Asylums*. In addition, you may have noted works by Franco Basaglia (1981), Frantz Fanon (2001), Thomas Scheff (2009), Gilles Deleuze and Félix Guattari (2000) and, the figure often credited with coining the term 'anti-psychiatry', David Cooper (1967).

Further reading

Gimenez J (2011) *Writing for Nursing and Midwifery Students*, 2nd edition. Basingstoke: Palgrave Macmillan.

This is a comprehensive introduction to academic writing for nursing students that includes, among other things, an extended discussion about avoiding plagiarism and using references in academic assignments.

Paul R & Elder L (2014) *Critical Thinking: Tools for taking charge of your professional and personal life*, 2nd edition. Upper Saddle River, NJ: Pearson Education.

Here you will find a comprehensive and stimulating work that discusses many aspects of critical thinking, including an examination of the 'universal intellectual standards' that are commonly employed to assess critical thinking and reflection.

Peck J & Coyle M (2012) *The Student's Guide to Writing: Spelling, punctuation and grammar*, 3rd edition. Basingstoke: Palgrave Macmillan.

A highly accessible and informative book that discusses how to incorporate correct spelling, punctuation and grammar into academic assignments and illustrates how doing so can add confidence, control and style to academic work.

Taylor DB (2013) *Writing Skills for Nursing and Midwifery Students*. London: Sage.

This book provides a comprehensive introduction to academic writing skills for nursing students and includes a detailed discussion of how to develop a writing style that is clear, concise and precise.

Useful websites

www.bbc.co.uk/skillswise/english

This is the BBC's Skillswise website that provides practical literacy skills for adults and includes a variety of information, resources and activities designed to develop competence with grammar, punctuation and spelling.

www.criticalthinking.org/pages/universal-intellectual-standards/527

Here you will find the website for the Centre for Critical Thinking and, in particular, an overview of commonly employed intellectual standards that are used to assess critical thinking and reflection.

Chapter 8
Critical evaluation

Chapter aims

By the end of this chapter you will be able to:

- understand the importance of **critical evaluation** for mental health nursing;
- identify a range of critically evaluative questions that can be used in mental health nursing;
- identify a variety of contexts in which to apply critically evaluative questions in mental health nursing.

Introduction

Case study

Amelia is currently at a mental health nursing conference with several other mental health nursing students in which she has been listening to a presentation about the future of the profession.

continued . . .

In concluding the presentation, the speaker suggested that the authority of mental health professionals is being called into question as never before, both by those who work within, and those who use, contemporary mental health services. Rather than simply accepting established ways of understanding and responding to mental health and distress, the speaker argued that it will be increasingly necessary for mental health nurses to evaluate critically all aspects of their mental health practice by subjecting it to 'rigorous and systematic questioning'. In discussing the presentation afterwards, Amelia and her colleagues are beginning to understand the need to develop their ability to engage in critical evaluation for both their university and clinical work. However, while she understands that this involves questioning the whole range of information to which she is being introduced during her mental health nursing programme, Amelia is unsure about the process of critical evaluation generally and, in particular, what 'rigorous and systematic' questions she ought to be asking.

Over the duration of your mental health nursing programme you will be introduced to a large amount of information in both the university setting and the clinical area. This will range from informal opinion, beliefs and speculation to formal research, theory and evidence and you will receive this information from a variety of sources, including lectures and tutorials, books and journal articles, presentations and conferences, professional guidance and peer discussions and, increasingly, through various forms of electronic media. However, rather than accepting this information uncritically, as you progress through your mental health nursing course you will be expected to subject that information to critical evaluation and consider its value for your mental health nursing practice. Indeed, an important aspect of becoming a professional, autonomous and accountable mental health nurse – and certainly in the context of the contemporary requirement to provide evidence-based practice in mental health nursing – is to be able to evaluate information in order to determine its worth for how you understand and respond to the needs of those who use mental health services. While a variety of guidelines, methods and frameworks have been proposed for critically evaluating information – and for critically appraising formal research in particular (Maltby *et al.* 2010; Greenhalgh 2014; Moule & Goodman 2014) – one of the most productive ways to engage in critical evaluation is to question rigorously and systematically the wide range of information to which you will be introduced or that you will access. However, while a variety of such critically evaluative questions have been proposed (Gimenez 2011; Woolliams *et al.* 2011), you may, like Amelia in the above case study, be unsure about the process of critical evaluation generally and, in particular, what rigorous and systematic questions you ought to be asking.

The purpose of this chapter is to introduce you to a series of questions that can be used to evaluate critically the large amount of information that you will encounter during your mental health nursing programme. In particular, it will discuss the importance of asking six critically evaluative questions of any piece of information to which you will be introduced, or that you may access, in both the university setting and the clinical area. First, we shall consider the need to ask about the content of the information and, in particular, to attempt to clarify what is being said; we shall then discuss the importance of asking where the information has come from and critically evaluating the source of that information; we shall also examine the importance of attempting to establish how the information has been produced and the particular means by which it has come to be known; then we shall discuss the need to ask who has produced the information and, closely associated with this, why that information has been produced; finally, we shall discuss the importance of establishing the age of the information and, in particular, of considering when the information was produced. By doing so, this chapter will assist you in developing the ability to apply these six critically evaluative questions consistently in the university setting and the clinical area; in particular, you will be encouraged to reflect upon and apply these six questions to the various forms of information that you will encounter during your mental health nursing programme and, subsequently, throughout your career as a mental health nurse.

What is being said?

Case study

Priya is a second-year mental health nursing student who is currently working on a university assignment in which she is required to provide a critical examination of the value of reflection for mental health nursing. In order to assist her with this, her tutor has recommended that she read a journal article that discusses the legitimacy of reflection as a means for generating knowledge within the context of evidence-based mental health nursing practice. However, somewhat to her annoyance, Priya is finding the article a particular challenge to read. So far on the mental health nursing programme she has found the reading material to be straightforward and has developed her ability to 'scan' books and articles quickly to find the information that she requires and, on other occasions, to 'skim' read such material in order to get a brief overview of its meaning. However, she is finding neither reading style particularly helpful for the article that her tutor has recommended, not least because of the terminology that is used throughout; for example, she has identified a variety of words and phrases that she has never encountered before, such as 'epistemology', 'critical realism', 'constructivism' and 'technical rationality'.

To evaluate critically any piece of information that you will encounter over the duration of your mental health nursing programme, it will be necessary to ask about the content of that information and, in particular, to attempt to determine what is being said. While you may often find this to be a relatively straightforward process, on other occasions, as Priya is experiencing in the above case study, it may prove to be more challenging. There can be many reasons why it might be difficult to determine the meaning of what is being said and these can range from the manner in which the information has been presented to the complexity of the material that you are attempting to understand. Indeed, a variety of issues in contemporary mental health care are inherently complex and, as you progress through your mental health nursing programme and are introduced to these issues, it may be necessary to work particularly hard in order to understand them. On occasions it may be sufficient, for example, to scan books and articles quickly to find the information that you require and to skim read such material in order to get a brief overview of the meaning; however, on other occasions this may not be sufficient and you may need to adopt other strategies to attempt to determine what is being said, such as reading in a more considered and methodical manner, clarifying words and phrases with which you are unfamiliar and discussing your understanding of the meaning of certain information with the understanding of others. In doing so, it is important to recognise that there may be disagreements about the meaning of the information that you are attempting to understand and, certainly with books and articles that introduce new concepts and theoretical frameworks, it may be possible to adopt significantly different perspectives on, and provide varying interpretations of, what is being said. However, while providing a new and innovative interpretation or 'reading' of a given text can be a considerable and highly valuable academic achievement, in seeking to determine the meaning of what is being said then it will be necessary to support your reading with considered and appropriate reference to the material that you are attempting to understand.

Activity 8.1   *Critical thinking*

At the beginning of his influential paper 'The myth of mental illness', Thomas Szasz (1983, p. 12) makes the following startling assertion: *My aim in this essay is to ask if there is such a thing as mental illness, and to argue that there is not.*

For this activity, access and read Szasz's (1983) paper and attempt to determine what is being said. You may find it necessary to read the paper in a considered and methodical manner and even perhaps read the paper more than once but, in doing so, it can be productive to read with a clear purpose or guiding question in mind. Therefore, as you read 'The myth of mental illness', consider if Szasz is proposing – as a brief reading of the opening of the paper appears to suggest – that the variety of problems and forms of distress that are commonly referred to as 'mental illness' do not exist or is he making a more subtle and nuanced claim?

An outline answer is provided at the end of the chapter.

Where does the information come from?

Case study

Frances and John have recently begun their mental health nursing programme and are discussing the use of the Mental Health Act 1983. Frances has been doing her own reading around the use of the Act and states that she has discovered that section 5(4), which is commonly referred to as 'the nurse's holding power', permits a registered mental health nurse to detain an informal hospital inpatient for up to nine hours if certain conditions are met. John is yet to do any detailed reading around the use of the Act but suggests that, while he is aware that the Act was amended in 2007, he thought that the nurse's holding power could only be used for up to six hours. However, Frances is adamant that it is nine hours; indeed, her apparent certainty is making John question his own

continued . . .

> *thoughts about the duration of the nurse's holding power and he therefore asks Frances where she has read this information so that he can access and verify it for himself. However, while Frances reiterates that she has read about the nurse's holding power recently, she says that she cannot remember exactly where she obtained the information, although she thinks it may have been on an internet forum about the use of the Act.*

In order to evaluate critically any piece of information that you will encounter in the university setting or the clinical area, it is not only necessary to ask what is being said but, like John in the above case study, it is productive to ask where that information has come from. Over the duration of your mental health nursing programme you will be introduced to and access information from a variety of sources and, in doing so, you ought to consider the extent to which those sources can be understood as credible, reliable and reputable. While it is possible to receive questionable information from established and credible sources, and to obtain correct information from what are considered unreliable and unsound sources, attempting to determine where the information has come from can often provide you with a strong indication of the quality of the material to which you are being introduced or that you are accessing. For example, articles in academic journals and books produced by an academic publisher – many of which are increasingly accessible online – will have been **peer-reviewed**. This means that the information contained within those journals and books will have been scrutinised by other professionals working in the same field as the author, the author's peers, and they will have judged that the information is accurate, credible and worthy of inclusion in the book or journal to which it has been submitted.

Less credible sources for academic and clinical purposes, however, include books that have been produced by commercial publishers. Although such books may be concerned with an academic subject, such as human anatomy, psychology or philosophy, they are commonly designed to inform (and often entertain) a general readership and not the academic community. Similarly, while a wide range of internet sources can provide a convenient and rapid means to obtain an initial overview of a topic, the information that you obtain from individual and business websites, open-source encyclopedias and personal blogs, online forums and other forms of social media should not be considered as credible sources of information for your university assignments and clinical practice. The primary reason for this is that, generally speaking, the information obtained from such sources will not have been subject to a formal peer-review process comparable to that provided by academic journals and book publishers, and so there are no assurances that the information obtained from such internet sources is complete, accurate or reliable. However, while you should be cautious about using internet sources to inform your university and clinical work, reputable sources can be found; these include, for example, the websites of governmental departments (e.g. the Department of Health), non-departmental public bodies (e.g. the National Institute for Health and Care Excellence), professional governing bodies (e.g. the Nursing and Midwifery Council) and the websites of respected charitable organisations (e.g. MIND, Rethink and the Mental Health Foundation).

Activity 8.2   *Decision making*

Consider the discussion between Frances and John in the above case study in which there is apparent disagreement and confusion about the duration of the nurse's holding power under section 5(4) of the Mental Health Act 1983. What credible information source could you refer to in order to determine satisfactorily the duration of the nurse's holding power?

An outline answer is provided at the end of the chapter.

How has the information been produced?

The information that you encounter over the duration of your mental health nursing programme will have been produced by a variety of means and, in order to evaluate that information critically, it can be productive to ask, and seek to determine, how that information has been produced. For example, some of that information may be the result of unreflective opinion, uninformed speculation and even stereotypical, discriminatory and exclusionary attitudes; in contrast, some information will have emerged as a consequence of critical reflection, informed debate and considered discussion about the theory and practice of contemporary mental health care; other forms of information will have been produced through rigorous critical thinking, systematic conceptual analysis and creative theoretical development; finally, some of the information that you encounter will be published, formal research that will have been produced through the employment of various **qualitative** and **quantitative research methodologies**. In considering the variety of means by which information is produced, and in assessing the respective value of those various means, it is important to recognise that, within the context of the contemporary requirement to provide evidence-based health care, information, evidence or knowledge that is produced by certain means has commonly been valued more highly than information, evidence or knowledge produced by other means. Indeed, while various hierarchies have been formulated that seek to determine the respective value of different forms of evidence, the majority place evidence obtained by using quantitative research methodologies (and **randomised controlled trials** in particular) as the most valuable, while expert opinion, clinical judgement and research conducted by qualitative means have often been placed towards the bottom, or omitted altogether, from such hierarchies (Guyatt *et al.* 1995; Geddes & Harrison 1997).

It is important to recognise, however, that 'hierarchies of evidence' that position information, evidence or knowledge produced by means of quantitative research as the most valuable have been subject to ongoing critical discussion and debate (Mantzoukas 2008; McKenna 2009; O'Halloran *et al.* 2010). While such debates are multifaceted and complex, an enduring critical concern is the degree to which such hierarchies, by prioritising quantitative research methodologies, devalue and even exclude the varied forms of information, evidence and knowledge that are claimed to be necessary to understand and respond to the range of issues that characterise contemporary mental health care. For example, if we are concerned with attempting to understand and determine the effectiveness of a specific intervention – such as the ability of a particular anti-psychotic drug to alleviate certain symptoms associated with a diagnosis of schizophrenia – then quantitative research methodologies may be the most valuable means to produce such information; however, if we are concerned with attempting to understand how people feel about something – such as why those who are prescribed an anti-psychotic drug may be reluctant to commence or, once commenced, continue taking that drug – then qualitative research methodologies may be more appropriate (Faulkner & Thomas 2002). Therefore, when critically evaluating the various means by which the information that you will encounter has been produced, it is necessary to consider if those means are suitable for the area of mental health care under discussion or if other means may be more appropriate. In doing so, you should recognise that the manner in which mental health nurses come to know the wide range of information, evidence and knowledge that underlies their practice is complex, diverse and multidimensional and the respective value of those various forms of knowing ought to be considered in the context in which they are being employed.

Concept summary: Fundamental patterns of knowing

The information, evidence and knowledge upon which nursing is based, and which serve as a rationale for nursing practice more generally, are complex, diverse and multidimensional. However, Barbara Carper (1978) proposed that the knowledge that nurses possess, and the manner in which such knowledge was produced, could be divided into four distinguishable, although interrelated and interdependent, 'forms' or 'patterns': (1) **empirical**; (2) **aesthetic**; (3) personal; and (4) ethical.

The empirical pattern of knowing – what Carper (1978) terms 'empirics' – refers to the knowledge that is obtained through observation and measurement and by conducting carefully controlled and replicable experiments to test hypotheses. From such experimental knowledge there is a development of abstract conceptual structures and 'general laws' and such activity is therefore characterised as the 'science' of nursing.

The aesthetic pattern of knowing refers to knowledge that often resists simple observation and measurement, such as the ability to empathise with others and establish therapeutic relationships more generally. Insofar as it is knowledge that is often developed through individual experience, and a creative, intuitive sense of how to proceed, it is commonly characterised as the 'art' of nursing.

The personal pattern of knowing refers to the knowledge of oneself, the ongoing ability to develop an awareness of one's strengths, weaknesses, values and assumptions. While this knowledge is identified by Carper (1978) as being potentially the most challenging to acquire, it is also essential for what is termed 'the therapeutic use of self' and an understanding of mental health nursing as an interpersonal process.

The ethical pattern of knowing refers to knowledge of the moral codes, ethical standards and professional values that characterise contemporary nursing. However, it also includes an ability to reflect critically upon, and responsibly apply, those standards in ethically problematic and ambiguous situations with a sensitivity to the requirements of being accountable for the ethical decisions that one makes.

Activity 8.3   *Reflection*

For this activity, carefully consider Carper's (1978) four fundamental patterns of knowing, identified above. As you do so, attempt to identify one instance when your mental health practice has been, or potentially could be, informed by the empirical pattern of knowing, the aesthetic pattern of knowing, the personal pattern of knowing and the ethical pattern of knowing.

As this activity is based on your own reflections, there is no outline answer at the end of the chapter.

Who has produced the information?

Case study

Adewale and his mental health nursing student colleagues are reflecting upon a tutorial that they have just received from Caroline, who describes herself as 'a survivor of the psychiatric system'. In particular, they are discussing what she had to say about the 'disempowering' consequences of receiving a diagnosis of schizophrenia and the 'dehumanising' and coercive practices that she maintains she was subject to as a consequence of that diagnosis. While Adewale and his colleagues found Caroline's critique of the field of health care into which they are entering both challenging and controversial, they all agree that it was a thought-provoking perspective on psychiatric diagnosis and contemporary mental health care more generally. In particular, Adewale is beginning to consider that he has, until now, given minimal consideration to the lived experience of receiving a diagnosis of schizophrenia; while he has acquired a body of 'professional knowledge' about that diagnosis – such as the range of so-called 'positive' and 'negative' symptoms – he is beginning to consider that he has yet to develop what Caroline referred to as 'the wisdom to recognise, respect and respond to the human being that exists prior to, and in spite of, any diagnostic category'.

In critically evaluating the wide range of information to which you will be introduced, or that you will access, during your mental health nursing programme, it is productive to consider who has produced that information. In particular, it is possible to gain an indication of the quality of the information that you will encounter by attempting to determine if the individual, group or organisation that has produced that information has any previous experience or expertise in the area of mental health care that is under consideration. However, it is important to recognise that, with the increased involvement of those who use mental health services in the provision, evaluation and development of those services, the notion of 'expertise' is becoming increasingly more inclusive. For example, while it is acknowledged that mental health nurses possess professional knowledge, experience and expertise, there is an increasing recognition that, like Caroline in the above case study, those who have used or who are currently using mental health services are to be understood as 'experts by experience', as individuals who possess insights into various aspects of contemporary mental health care – such as the lived experience of receiving a diagnosis of schizophrenia – that may not be immediately available to mental health professionals. However, while attempting to determine who has produced the information that you will encounter can provide you with an indication of its quality, you should be cautious about accepting or rejecting any information exclusively on the basis of who has produced or who is communicating that information. Indeed, it is possible to receive questionable information from those who are considered experts in contemporary mental health care and to obtain insightful, stimulating and valuable information from those who are thought to have minimal knowledge, experience and expertise. Therefore, while it is important to recognise and respect the expertise of those who are considered authorities in a given area of contemporary mental health care, it is necessary primarily to attend to the content of what is being said without being overawed by, or dismissive of, the status of the individual, group or organisation that has produced or is communicating such information.

Activity 8.4   *Evidence-based practice and research*

The Scottish Recovery Network is a non-profit organisation working in Scotland and beyond that aims to promote and support recovery from mental distress. A central aspect of its work involves conducting research that aims to listen and learn from the experiences of those who describe themselves as recovered, or recovering, from mental distress.

For this activity, access, read and consider the document *Journeys of Recovery* (**www.scottish recovery.net/View-document-details/81-Journeys-of-Recovery.html**), which provides 12 accounts, stories or 'narratives' of the lived experience of recovery. As you read the narratives of those who have recovered, or are recovering, from mental distress, consider if they provide you with information, insights and knowledge about recovery that you may not have been able to obtain from those who have not had such an experience.

As this activity is based on your own research and reflection, there is no outline answer at the end of the chapter.

Why has the information been produced?

In order to evaluate critically the information that you will encounter during your mental health nursing programme, it is not only productive to ask who has produced that information but, closely associated with this, to consider why they have produced that information. In doing so, it is necessary to recognise that there may be multiple reasons why an individual, group or organisation may have produced a given piece of information or may be presenting that information in a particular way. For example, it may be a consequence of a desire to improve the quality of mental health care and, in turn, the experiences of those who use mental health services; it may be the result of uncertainty over some aspect of the theory or practice of contemporary mental health nursing and a wish to explore, and attempt to address, that uncertainty; alternatively, it may be a consequence of a decision to question, critique or even discredit the knowledge, information or opinions offered by others; finally, it may be because it is in the interests of an individual, group or organisation to produce a certain piece of information, or present that information in a particular way, and doing so is likely to result in some form of personal, professional or financial gain.

The information to which you will be introduced, or that you might access, during your mental health nursing programme may therefore have emerged as a consequence of a variety of motives, interests and affiliations. However, when attempting to determine why a given piece of information has been produced, or has been presented in a particular way, it is important to recognise that having motives, interests and affiliations is not, in and of itself, sufficient to invalidate that piece of information. Indeed, not only are intentions, interests and affiliations an acceptable, and arguably unavoidable, aspect of working within contemporary mental health care, but they can also be powerful, motivating factors that can direct and sustain the continued production and communication of insightful, stimulating and valuable information. In the above case study, for example, it may be that Caroline's negative experiences of contemporary mental health care services have motivated her to share her experiences with mental health nursing students and this, in turn, has motivated Adewale and his colleagues to begin to reflect critically upon the implications of those experiences for their mental health practice. Therefore, when asking why a particular piece of information has been produced, or has been presented in a particular way, it is not sufficient solely to attempt to determine what motives, interests and affiliations may have influenced the production of that information; rather, it is also necessary to ask whether those motives, interests and affiliations have 'unduly influenced' the production and presentation of that information and, in particular, have led to information being produced and presented in a way that is likely to misrepresent, mislead or deceive.

Activity 8.5 — *Critical thinking*

Owing to concerns about the influence of authors' motives, interests and affiliations on the production of information, academic journals commonly require authors to make a 'declaration of competing interests', which is often included in the article itself. In doing so, authors are required to declare if they have any motives, affiliations or interests that might have led them, whether knowingly or otherwise, to produce information that is likely to misrepresent, mislead or deceive those who encounter such information.

- What motives, interests or affiliations might authors have that could lead them, whether knowingly or otherwise, to produce information that is likely to misrepresent, mislead or deceive?

An outline answer is provided at the end of the chapter.

When was the information produced?

Case study

Jessica and Dean, two second-year mental health nursing students, are currently conducting a joint literature search for an assignment that is concerned with spirituality and mental health care. In doing so, Dean states that he has found a book that, while it appears challenging, might be relevant insofar as it appears to discuss spirituality in the context of interpersonal relationships and, in particular, that which it refers to as the 'I–Thou' encounter. Listening to Dean's brief description of the work, Jessica agrees that it may be relevant for their assignment and, as part of the inclusion and exclusion criteria for their literature search, asks when it was published. Dean states that, although he has an edition of the work that was published three years ago, the first English translation of the book was published over 75 years ago. Jessica suggests that, while it seems to be relevant for the area of mental health care that they are investigating, they will not be able to use the book because, as she understands it, they are only allowed to use material that has been published in the last ten years.

As you may already be aware, within the context of the contemporary requirement to provide evidence-based mental health care, it is necessary to practise in accordance with *the best available evidence* (Tee & Lathlean 2012). A central aspect of this requirement is to ensure that the evidence, knowledge and information that guide your mental health practice are the best that are currently available and have not been superseded by more recent evidence, knowledge and information. In order to evaluate critically the wide range of information that you will encounter during your mental health nursing programme, it is therefore productive to consider, like Jessica in the above case study, when that information was produced. However, as we have already discussed, the evidence, information and knowledge that are said to be necessary to understand and respond to the range of issues that characterise contemporary mental health care are complex, diverse and multidimensional; while it is an established principle that such information ought to be the best that is currently available, it is possible that in some areas of contemporary mental health care the age of the best information that is currently available may exceed, for example, the criteria set by Jessica in the above case study.

While it is commonly supposed that more recent information is, by that fact alone, superior to older information, it is important to recognise the rich heritage of thought that characterises the varied disciplines that either directly or indirectly inform contemporary mental health nursing. Indeed, the knowledge that can be found within that heritage can be valuable for enabling us to understand and respond to the complexities of the present and, certainly in academic settings, the ability to recover, reinvigorate and resituate such knowledge by bringing it to bear on contemporary issues in mental health care can be a highly productive activity. Accordingly, in asking and attempting to determine when the information that you will encounter during your mental health nursing programme was produced, you should be cautious of discarding it simply on the basis of its age; for some areas of study in mental health care it will be appropriate to do so but in other areas, such as that being investigated by Jessica and Dean in the above case study, discarding information on the basis of age will inhibit your discovery of information that may potentially be of value for both your university and clinical work. Therefore, in addition to considering when the information that you will encounter during your mental health nursing programme was produced, it will also be productive to evaluate critically whether such information may be valuable for the particular area under discussion and whether it can enable you to understand and respond to the varied complexities that characterise contemporary mental health care.

Activity 8.6 *Evidence-based practice and research*

As you are probably already aware, cognitive behavioural therapy is widely recognised as the contemporary psychological treatment of choice for a variety of forms of mental distress. Indeed, the evidence base for its effectiveness in treating people with depression and anxiety established the economic case for the Improving Access to Psychological Therapies programme, and this was reflected in the initial intention of that programme to establish a 'strong core' of cognitive behavioural therapists and psychological wellbeing practitioners across the UK (DH 2011b). However, the two most significant thinkers on the development of cognitive behavioural therapy, Albert Ellis and Aaron Beck, both acknowledged the profound influence of a particular school of ancient Western philosophy on that therapeutic approach.

For this activity, attempt to discover which school of ancient Western philosophy is acknowledged as underpinning cognitive behavioural therapy. It is a school of philosophy that emerged in Athens around 300 BCE and advocated a variety of psychological techniques and exercises that are said to be consistent with contemporary cognitive behavioural therapy (Robertson 2010). In addition, attempt to determine two major exponents of that ancient school of philosophy.

An outline answer is provided at the end of the chapter.

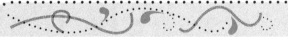

Chapter summary

In this chapter we have discussed the importance of being able to evaluate critically the large amount of information that you will encounter during your mental health nursing programme. Being able to engage in critical evaluation is a significant skill that will greatly enhance your ability to become a professional, autonomous and accountable mental health nurse who is able to evaluate information in order to determine its worth for how you understand and respond to the needs of those who use mental health services. While a variety of guidelines, methods and frameworks have been proposed for critically evaluating information, we have suggested that it is productive to ask six questions of any piece of information to which you will be introduced, or that you may access, in both the university setting and the clinical area. In particular, we have discussed the need to ask about the

continued . . .

content of the information and, specifically, to attempt to clarify what is being said; we have then considered the need to ask where the information has come from and to evaluate critically the source of that information; we have also examined the importance of attempting to establish how the information has been produced and the particular means by which it has come to be known; in addition, we have discussed the need to ask who has produced the information and, closely associated with this, to attempt to determine why that information has been produced; finally, we have examined the need to establish the age of the information and, in particular, to consider when the information was produced. By doing so, this chapter has encouraged you to reflect upon and apply these six critically evaluative questions to the various forms of information that you will encounter during your mental health nursing programme and, subsequently, throughout your career as a mental health nurse.

Activities: brief outline answers

Activity 8.1 Critical thinking

Despite his explicit claim that there is no such thing as mental illness at the beginning of his influential paper 'The myth of mental illness', Thomas Szasz (1983) is not suggesting that the variety of problems and forms of distress that are commonly referred to as 'mental illness' do not exist. As he makes clear, *While I maintain that mental illnesses do not exist, I obviously do not imply or mean that the social and psychological occurrences to which this label is attached also do not exist* (Szasz 1983, p. 21). Instead, those varied forms of distress that are referred to as mental illnesses are to be understood as *problems in living* that not only arise as a consequence of the stress, strain and disharmony that are said to occur at all levels of human relations, but also because of the contemporary challenge of attempting to give purpose, direction and meaning to one's life (Szasz 1983, pp. 21–2; Roberts 2007). To refer to those problems in living as mental illnesses – to understand the very real personal, social and **existential problems** that people experience as illnesses or diseases that can be resolved by medical means – is to conceal the real character of those problems. Therefore, Szasz (1983, pp. 21–3) proposes that the application of medical terminology to those problems is inappropriate and the notion of mental illness is to be understood as a *disguise*, a *social tranquillizer* or a *myth* that serves to obscure the personal, social and existential character of the problems in living that many contemporary people confront.

Activity 8.2 Decision making

In order to determine satisfactorily the duration of the nurse's holding power, and resolve the apparent disagreement between Frances and John, there are a number of credible sources to which you could refer. The most obvious is the Mental Health Act 1983 itself (which is available online and to download at **www. legislation.gov.uk/ukpga/1983/20/contents**). However, in order to assist health care professionals to understand and implement the Act in a legal, safe and responsible manner, the Department of Health (2015a) publishes a Code of Practice to which you could also refer (available online and to download at **www.gov.uk/government/publications/code-of-practice-mental-health-act-1983**). In addition, you could access the *Reference Guide to the Mental Health Act 1983* (DH 2015b) that is designed to complement the Code of Practice in assisting health care professionals to understand and implement the Act (also available online at **www.gov.uk/government/publications/mental-health-act-1983-reference-guide**). While the foregoing should be your definitive sources to determine the duration of the nurse's holding power, and any other issues relating to the Act, you may initially find academic books aimed at mental health nurses and other health care professionals more accessible and a number of reputable academic books are available to enable you to develop your understanding of, and your responsibilities under, the Mental Health Act 1983 (e.g. Barber *et al.* 2012; Murphy & Wales 2013).

Activity 8.5 Critical thinking

While there are potentially a variety of motives, affiliations and interests that might lead an author, either knowingly or otherwise, to produce misleading or deceitful information, you may have identified that the main interests are concerned with personal, professional and financial gain. For example, when making a declaration of competing interests, authors are required to declare if they have received funding in order to produce the information, if they are associated or employed by a company that may benefit from the publication of the information or if they are expected to receive financial gain as a consequence of producing the information or because they have presented that information in a particular way.

Activity 8.6 Evidence-based practice and research

Contemporary cognitive behavioural therapy can predominantly be understood as emerging from the work of Albert Ellis, the pioneer of rational emotive behaviour therapy, and Aaron Beck, the originator of cognitive therapy. While acknowledging the influence of Buddhist and Taoist thought on their work, they both also acknowledged the influence of ancient Western philosophy on their respective approaches and, in particular, the influence of that school of ancient philosophy called Stoicism (Ellis 1962; Beck *et al.* 1979). In attempting to identify two major exponents of Stoicism, you may have identified a wide variety of figures, including Zeno of Citium, who is recognised as founding Stoicism in Athens around 300 BCE, and also Cleanthes and then Chrysippus, who were the subsequent leaders of that school of philosophy; however, Stoicism also flourished in ancient Rome and you may have identified that major Stoic thinkers during this period included Seneca, Epictetus and the Roman Emperor Marcus Aurelius (Sellars 2006).

Further reading

Aveyard H, Sharp P & Woolliams M (2015) *A Beginner's Guide to Critical Thinking and Writing in Health and Social Care*, 2nd edition. Maidenhead: Open University Press.

This is an accessible introduction to critical thinking and writing in health and social care settings that includes, among other things, a discussion about how to find and evaluate information for health and social care practice.

Cottrell S (2011) *Critical Thinking Skills: Developing effective analysis and argument*, 2nd edition. Basingstoke: Palgrave Macmillan.

Although not specific to health care, this book provides a comprehensive account of how to develop a range of critical thinking skills, including the ability to clarify the content of information and evaluate the credibility of the source of that information.

Ellis P (ed) (2013) *Evidence-Based Practice in Nursing*. London: Sage/Learning Matters.

Here you will find an accessible introduction to evidence-based practice in nursing that includes an extended discussion about how to evaluate critically various forms of research and assess their value for nursing practice.

Greenhalgh T (2014) *How to Read a Paper: The basics of evidence-based medicine*, 5th edition. Chichester: John Wiley.

An established and comprehensive work that discusses the rationale for evidence-based medicine and provides a detailed account of how to search for, clarify the content of and systematically appraise published research.

Useful websites

www.casp-uk.net

Here you will find the website for the Critical Appraisal Skills Programme that provides information, resources and training on how to evaluate critically various forms of health care research.

Chapter 9
Critical writing

Chapter aims

By the end of this chapter you will be able to:

• identify the need to engage in critical writing for your mental health nursing programme;
• understand how to produce a systematic, coherent and convincing piece of critical writing;
• identify the central structural elements necessary to produce a systematic, coherent and convincing piece of critical writing.

Introduction

Case study

Ruth is a second-year mental health nursing student and is currently working on a university assignment in which she is required, in no more than 2,000 words, to 'Critically discuss the ethical justification for the use of compulsory powers under the Mental Health Act 1983'. Over the course of the

continued . . .

> *module for which the assignment has been set, Ruth remembers several lectures in which a variety of*
> *ethically problematic issues in mental health nursing, and contemporary mental health care more gen-*
> *erally, were discussed. In particular, she recalls the manner in which those issues were situated within*
> *the context of what is referred to as 'principlism', an approach to health care ethics that employs a*
> *variety of general principles such as autonomy,* **beneficence, non-maleficence** *and justice. However,*
> *although she intends to address the assignment question by employing this principlist approach, and*
> *while she already has extensive lecture notes on the approach that she feels will be relevant for her work,*
> *she is unsure how to organise all of that material in order to produce a systematic, coherent and con-*
> *vincing piece of critical writing.*

Over the course of your mental health nursing programme you will be required to engage in various forms of academic writing such as case study reports, journal article reviews and reflective analyses of your mental health practice. However, one of the most challenging forms of academic writing that you will be expected to carry out – not least because it demands the employment of a variety of higher-level thinking skills – is that which is variously referred to as analytical, argumentative or critical writing: writing in which you demonstrate your ability to engage critically with the diverse, challenging and often contested issues that characterise contemporary mental health care. In the previous two chapters we have examined the importance of critically evaluating the wide range of information that you will encounter during your mental health nursing programme and of working in accordance with the variety of academic standards against which your university assignments can be assessed. In developing such capabilities – as well as the various intellectual skills and emotional attributes that are associated with critical thinking and reflection and which were examined in the first part of this book – you will already be developing your ability to engage in critical writing for your university assignments. However, in addition to developing the capability to engage in analysis and reasoning, to appraise critically various forms of information and to add detail, depth and breadth to your university work, the challenge that critical writing presents is how to bring all of those varied elements together in a systematic, coherent and convincing manner. Indeed, while you may have conducted excellent preparatory work for your assignments and while you may have many interesting ideas that you wish to express in your critical writing, it has been suggested that, like Ruth in the above case study, many students find it a particular challenge to produce coherent, systematic and 'well-disciplined' essays that reflect the excellent preparatory work that they have conducted and the stimulating ideas that they have to communicate (Peck & Coyle 2012).

The purpose of this chapter is to introduce you to the notion of critical writing and to enable you to consider how you can begin to develop your ability to engage in that form of writing for your university assignments. In particular, it will propose that, in order to produce consistently high-quality critical writing, it is productive to attend to the structure of your work which, in turn, will assist you in organising and expressing the content of that work in a systematic, coherent and convincing manner. A variety of suggestions for organising and facilitating academic writing have been proposed, and for writing on university nursing programmes in particular (Gimenez 2011; Price & Harrington 2013; Taylor 2013); indeed, it is likely that your university has produced its own guidance on academic writing which you should access, read and consider carefully. However, throughout this chapter we shall be discussing that which has been referred to as 'the rule of three', which is a way of understanding your critical writing, and indeed any other form of writing that you may conduct during your mental health nursing programme, in terms of a three-part structure (Peck & Coyle 2012). After introducing the notion of the rule of three, this chapter will then examine each of the sections that comprise that three-part structure and how each section leads to the next to form an integrated whole that is characterised by a clear direction and a systematic, logical progression. As with all of the skills and attributes associated with critical thinking and reflection, the ability to produce coherent and convincing critical writing will take time, practice and patience to develop; however, throughout this chapter you will be encouraged to reflect upon, and work in accordance with, the rule of three in order to begin to develop your ability to produce consistently high-quality critical writing for your mental health nursing programme.

The rule of three

Case study

Although Ruth has attempted to begin writing her assignment, she is continuing to find it a particular challenge to organise her preparatory material and has therefore decided to seek the advice of her tutor. After considering her difficulties with ordering her critical writing and the structure of her essay more generally, Ruth's tutor suggests that she might benefit from thinking about her assignment in terms of the rule of three. Ruth has never heard of this before and states that, rather than spending time thinking about the structure of her assignment, she would rather focus on the content of the essay and, in particular, begin writing. However, her tutor reassures her that the time she spends thinking about the structure of her critical writing will also assist her with ordering the content of that writing. Ruth therefore says that she will attempt to follow the rule of three for this assignment if it will help her to organise her notes, express her ideas more clearly and, hopefully, improve the grades that she receives for her university assignments.

As you are probably already aware, for every essay that you write on your mental health nursing programme you will be required to provide an introduction and a conclusion to that work. However, the challenge that a piece of critical writing presents is what to put in between that introduction and conclusion and, as Ruth in the above case study is attempting to address, how to organise that material in a structured, systematic and coherent manner. In order to help you do so, it is productive to employ that which is commonly referred to as the rule of three in which your critical writing can be thought of in terms of an equally distributed three-part structure, as being comprised of three equal sections or three balanced developmental stages (Peck & Coyle 2012). In particular, the first section of that three-part structure requires you to establish what the area or issue under investigation is going to be, to 'set the scene' or 'lay the foundations' for what you are going to discuss critically; in the second section of that three-part structure you are required to develop the central features of the area under investigation, to 'move the discussion along', and do so by adding further detail, depth and breadth of thought to your critical writing;

finally, the third section of the three-part structure that characterises the rule of three requires you, as it were, to 'arrive somewhere', to bring the varied elements of your investigation together in such a way that you are able to reach some form of conclusion, however provisional or tentative it may be.

By enabling you to consider your critical writing in terms of a three-part structure, the rule of three therefore provides you with a framework within which you can organise and express your ideas and, importantly, introduces a sense of direction and development to your critical writing. Indeed, it has been suggested that one of the main advantages of using the rule of three for writing essays at a university level, and certainly for writing essays in which you are required to investigate and engage critically with a particular issue, is that it adheres to the character or 'logic' of all arguments in which propositions are introduced, the argument is developed and a conclusion is reached (Peck & Coyle 2012). However, in order to ensure that your writing possesses such a systematic, logical and proportional progression in which equal attention is given to each section of its three-part structure, it can be productive to consider the division of your work in numerical terms. For example, in the case study above, Ruth is permitted 2,000 words for her assignment and one way of ensuring that it possesses three sections in which each section receives equal consideration is to allocate 100 words for a brief introduction to the area under investigation and 100 words for a similarly brief summary or conclusion to that work. As illustrated in Table 9.1, doing so will leave Ruth with 1,800 words which, using the rule of three, can be divided into three sections of 600 words while each section can, in turn, be further divided into three paragraphs of 200 words.

Essay sections	Words
Introduction	100
Section 1: 'Set the scene'	600 (3 paragraphs of 200 words)
Section 2: 'Develop the discussion'	600 (3 paragraphs of 200 words)
Section 3: 'Arrive somewhere'	600 (3 paragraphs of 200 words)
Conclusion	100
Total	**2,000**

Table 9.1: A numerical division of a 2,000-word essay using the rule of three

When considering the division of your critical writing by such numerical means it is important to recognise, as we shall discuss below, that it is possible to add a degree of flexibility and variation to the rule of three in order to suit your particular academic purposes. However, the advantage of employing such numerical means when applying the rule of three to your critical writing is that it enables you to divide a discussion of any area or issue in contemporary mental health care into three equal sections, with each section representing a proportional stage in your critical discussion and each paragraph of those individual stages representing a clear progression in that discussion. In doing so, the rule of three can enable you to address many of the common problems that you may confront when engaging in critical writing and, indeed, any writing that you are required to conduct during your mental health nursing programme. In particular, it can help you to avoid producing disorganised essays in which your critical writing lacks a clear direction and a logical progression; it can also help to prevent critical writing that lacks balance in which, for example, there are unnecessarily long paragraphs that may obscure the point being developed or, conversely, paragraphs that are too short and only permit cursory, superficial claims to be made; finally, the three-part structure that characterises the rule of three can help save you a significant amount of time insofar as both the overall structure, and the elements that comprise that structure, are already determined and therefore allow you to concentrate on developing the content of your critical writing.

Activity 9.1 — *Decision making*

By providing you with a framework that determines the overall shape and direction of your critical writing, the rule of three enables you to focus your attention on the content of each section of your work and, in turn, each paragraph of those individual sections. However, while providing you with an overarching three-part structure within which you can organise and express your ideas, it is important to recognise that it is possible to add a degree of flexibility and variation to that structure if it is necessary to do so for your particular academic purposes.

For example, we have suggested that the 2,000-word assignment that Ruth in the above case study has been set can be divided, using the rule of three, into three sections of 600 words, with each section further divided into three paragraphs of 200 words. For this activity, consider how else you could numerically divide Ruth's 2,000-word essay into an overarching three-part structure that gives equal consideration to each of its three sections.

An outline answer is provided at the end of the chapter.

Introducing the work

Before we examine each of the individual sections that comprise the three-part structure that characterises the rule of three, it is productive first to discuss the introduction to any piece of critical writing. At its most fundamental level, your introduction is that which should clearly and concisely inform the reader what is the issue or area of mental health care that you are going to discuss critically and, importantly, how you are going to conduct that discussion. The most straightforward way to achieve this is by proposing to address the particular essay question that you have been set and, having begun to think about the content of your work in accordance with the rule of three, briefly outlining what you are going to do in each of the three sections. However, it is important to note that, while the employment of the rule of three may provide you with a more or less detailed notion of what you are going to examine in each of those three sections, it may not be until you have completed those sections that you are clear about what it is that you have discussed; indeed, while it may seem logical to begin your introduction first, you may find, somewhat paradoxically, that it is more productive to finalise your introduction after you have completed the three main sections that comprise your piece of critical writing.

While proposing to address the essay question that you have been set, and outlining how you are going to address that particular question, is an acceptable and adequate introduction to your critical writing, it is possible to introduce your critical discussion in a more sophisticated manner. That is, you can provide an introduction to your work that stimulates the interests of your readers and, in particular, does so by emphasising the importance of providing a critical discussion of the area of mental health care about which you are going to write. There are a variety of ways in which you can do this and you should practise incorporating these into your writing to produce more sophisticated introductions to your work: for example, one of the most effective techniques is to begin with a bold point, significant feature or arresting fact about contemporary mental health care and how this point, feature or fact necessitates the critical discussion that you are proposing to provide; in contrast, you may have discovered that there is an apparent absence of critical analyses in the literature about the area that you are proposing to investigate and you can suggest that your work will begin to address this apparent omission; alternatively, an effective way to introduce your critical writing is to draw attention to how your critical discussion can help to explore, clarify and even potentially address an enduring dilemma or problem in contemporary mental health care.

Activity 9.2   *Evidence-based practice and research*

In the above case study, the assignment that Ruth has been set requires her to discuss critically the ethical justification for the use of compulsory powers under the Mental Health Act 1983. In order to provide an introduction to her critical writing that stimulates the interests of her readers and highlights the importance of her critical discussion, Ruth could begin by drawing attention to a significant point, fact or feature about the contemporary use of those compulsory powers.

For this activity, go to the website for the Care Quality Commission – the independent body that is responsible, among other things, for monitoring the use of the Mental Health Act 1983 – and access its most recent annual report into the use of the Act (**www.cqc.org.uk/content/mental-health-act-annual-report-201314**). In particular, find out how often the Mental Health Act 1983 was used during 2013–2014, along with any other significant features about the use of those compulsory powers that could be included in the introduction to Ruth's critical writing.

An outline answer is provided at the end of the chapter.

Section 1: 'Set the scene'

Case study

*Having discussed the application of the rule of three to her assignment with her tutor – and having supported this with her own reading about dividing her critical writing into three balanced stages that have a clear direction and a logical progression – Ruth understands that in the first section she is required to set the scene for her critical discussion. In thinking about what to include in this section, she has therefore decided to provide an overview of principlism as an approach to health care ethics and, in particular, to introduce, define and discuss the notions of autonomy, beneficence, non-maleficence and justice. However, over the course of the module for which the assignment has been set, she recalls the suggestion that what made many practices in contemporary mental health care ethically problematic, including the use of compulsory powers under the Mental Health Act 1983, was the manner in which they could be understood as instances of **paternalism**. Therefore, in addition to the four main principles that are commonly associated with principlism, she has also decided to introduce, define and discuss the notion of paternalism in section one of her critical writing and, in particular, to situate all of these notions in the context of contemporary mental health nursing.*

After the introduction to your critical writing, the first section of the three-part structure that characterises the rule of three requires you to establish what the area or issue under investigation is going to be, to set the scene or lay the foundations for what you are going to discuss critically. A productive way to begin to do this is, like Ruth in the above case study, to introduce, define and discuss what underpins your critical discussion, such as the significant concepts, the theoretical framework or the particular approach that you are adopting in your critical writing. In doing so, it is important to demonstrate your knowledge and comprehension of what underpins your work and a common, established way to do this is, for example, to define the key terms or significant concepts that you will be using to inform your critical discussion. However, as we noted in Chapter 7, if you display your knowledge and comprehension by simply listing, describing and repeating what you have been taught over the course of a particular module, or over the duration of your mental health nursing programme more generally, then your work is likely to be considered as superficial and lacking in depth.

While you are expected to employ what you have been taught over the course of a particular module, and while it is important that you make reference to the available literature when providing definitions of the key terms and concepts that inform your work, it is possible to display your knowledge and comprehension of that which underpins your critical writing in a more sophisticated and convincing manner. For example, you can paraphrase an existing definition of a key term in your own words in order to demonstrate that you have reflected upon and understood the meaning of that term; in addition, you can discuss the varying definitions of a single concept in order to demonstrate your awareness of the complex, multidimensional and possibly contested character of that concept before settling on a provisional definition for your critical writing; finally, insofar as the definitions of the key terms and concepts that underpin your critical discussion are likely to be broad, general and abstract statements, a productive way to display your knowledge and comprehension is to provide actual, 'concrete' clinical instances of those terms or concepts and, by doing so, demonstrate examples in the context of contemporary mental health nursing.

Activity 9.3   *Critical thinking*

In health care ethics, paternalism has been defined as the practice on the part of people in positions of power and authority of limiting, obstructing or overriding the freedom, autonomy and preferences of other people; in order to limit such freedom, it has been suggested that paternalistic acts in health care typically involve a variety of means, including force, coercion, deception and the manipulation of information (Beauchamp 2000; Beauchamp & Childress 2001).

For this activity, demonstrate your knowledge and comprehension of that general definition of paternalism by situating it in a clinical context. In particular, provide three clinical examples of what could be understood as paternalistic acts, practices or policies in contemporary mental health care.

An outline answer is provided at the end of the chapter.

Section 2: 'Develop the discussion'

Case study

After setting the scene in the first section of her assignment by discussing the notion of paternalism in the context of contemporary mental health care, along with the main notions associated with principlism as an approach to health care ethics, Ruth understands that in the second section she is required to develop her critical discussion. In doing so, she has decided to detail how those notions relate to one another by suggesting that the use of compulsory powers under the Mental Health Act 1983 is paternalistic and ethically problematic because it can be understood as being in conflict with a person's autonomy, as limiting the freedom and preferences of those who come into contact with mental health services. However, in this section of her work, Ruth also intends to discuss and evaluate the established argument that acts of paternalism in mental health care are often justified by invoking the notions of beneficence and non-maleficence; that the use of compulsory powers, for example, will ensure good and prevent harm occurring to the person whose autonomy, freedom and preferences have been restricted by those powers.

Having set the scene in the first section of your critical writing, the second section of the three-part structure that characterises the rule of three requires you to move your discussion along, to develop the critical discussion that you began in the first section of your assignment. There are a variety of ways in which you can develop your discussion and, in part, this will be determined by the character of the particular area or issue of contemporary mental health care that you are investigating. For example, like Ruth in the above case study, developing your discussion can involve a greater degree of analysis about what underpins your critical discussion, a consideration of how the key terms or concepts relate to one another or how the theoretical framework or particular approach that you are adopting can be applied to the area of mental health care under consideration. However, irrespective of the particular area or issue under investigation, the requirement to move your discussion along in the second section of your critical writing will invariably mean that you will adopt a position or a perspective in relation to that which is under investigation and this will require you to identify, evaluate and even formulate arguments that may be relevant for your work.

While developing your critical discussion will require you to identify, evaluate and even formulate arguments in order to adopt a position in relation to that which is being investigated, it may not be immediately clear to you what an argument is. Indeed, there are a variety of definitions, of varying complexity, about what constitutes an argument as well as numerous suggestions about how to identify, construct and evaluate arguments and it will be productive for you to access, read and carefully consider these varying accounts (Weston 2009; Cottrell 2011; Swatridge 2014). However, it has been suggested that at its most fundamental level an argument consists of both a claim that something is the case and the reason that is given for why that claim ought to be accepted (Taylor 2013; Wallace & Wray 2013). As we discussed in Chapter 1, there may be multiple reasons given for why a particular claim ought to be accepted and this can range from uninformed speculation and unreflective opinion to rigorous critical thinking and reference to established or new research. Therefore, the particular challenge that you confront in moving the discussion along in your critical writing, and critically engaging with arguments in particular, is to begin to develop the ability to appraise the quality of the reasons given for why a particular claim ought, or ought not, to be accepted.

Activity 9.4 — *Team working*

In the above case study, Ruth is developing her critical discussion by identifying and attempting to evaluate the argument for the use of compulsory powers under the Mental Health Act 1983. In particular, such powers are often justified by invoking the notions of beneficence and non-maleficence, by proposing that the use of those powers ensures good and prevents harm occurring to the person who is subject to those powers or, in addition, prevents that person from harming others.

Consider this argument for the use of compulsory powers in contemporary mental health care and, with your colleagues, discuss whether the use of those powers, despite restricting a person's autonomy, is justified with reference to beneficence and non-maleficence. In particular, consider whether it is sufficient to justify the use of compulsory powers under the Mental Health Act 1983 by suggesting that they ensure good and prevent harm or whether further reasons are necessary to support an argument for the use of those powers.

An outline answer is provided at the end of the chapter.

Section 3: 'Arrive somewhere'

Case study

While Ruth has set the scene for her critical discussion in the first section of her assignment, and has moved that discussion along in the second section, she understands that in the third and final section of her critical writing it is necessary to reach some form of conclusion. In considering this, she has decided to propose that principlism is, in the main, a productive approach by which to analyse the ethical justification for the use of compulsory powers under the Mental Health Act 1983. However, after conducting more extensive reading around the topic, Ruth has discovered that there are a number of alternative approaches to health care ethics and that these can be understood as highlighting some of the potential limitations of principlism. While she recognises that she will be unable to consider all of those alternative approaches in section three of her assignment, Ruth has decided to include a discussion of what is referred to as 'the ethics of care'; in particular, she intends to discuss how that approach to health care ethics provides an account of the potential limitations of principlism as an approach to understanding the ethical issues surrounding the use of compulsory powers in contemporary mental health care.

The third and final section of the three-part structure that characterises the rule of three requires you to arrive somewhere, to bring the varied elements of your critical discussion together in such a way that you are able to reach some form of conclusion. It is important to note, however, that the requirement to arrive somewhere and reach some form of conclusion does not mean that you are expected somehow to 'definitively resolve', or provide a 'conclusive solution' to, the issue or area of mental health care that is under investigation. As we have suggested, many of the critical issues that characterise contemporary mental health care are challenging, complex and multidimensional and they often resist attempts to be reduced to a set of easy answers and simplistic solutions. For example, in considering the ethical justification for acts of paternalism in health care, of which the use of compulsory powers under the Mental Health Act 1983 can be understood as an instance, Beauchamp and Childress (2001, p. 187) – the major exponents of the principlist approach to health care ethics – have not only suggested that *It is a messy and complicated problem, and coherence in our judgements is difficult to achieve*, but have also noted that *Developing a position on paternalism requires appreciating the limits of principles and the need to give them additional content.*

While the rule of three requires you to reach some form of conclusion in the third section of your critical discussion, it is therefore likely to have a provisional or tentative character which acknowledges the complexity of the area of mental health care under investigation. One of the most productive ways in which you can provide such a conclusion is not only to acknowledge the strengths of the particular approach or perspective that you have adopted in your critical writing but also to acknowledge its potential limitations. For example, in the above case study, Ruth has reached the conclusion that principlism can broadly be understood as a productive framework by which to analyse the ethical justification for the use of compulsory powers under the Mental

Health Act 1983; however, she is providing a provisional or tentative conclusion that highlights the complexity of that issue insofar as she has also decided to discuss the potential limitations of principlism by drawing upon an alternative approach to health care ethics. Indeed, in identifying the complexity that is characteristic of many critical issues in mental health care, it can be a sign of academic sophistication and maturity to acknowledge the existence of a variety of approaches and perspectives on any given issue and, in doing so, to acknowledge that those alternative approaches and perspectives may provide valuable opportunities for further critical investigation into the issue or area of mental health care under consideration.

Activity 9.5   *Evidence-based practice and research*

In the above case study, Ruth has identified a number of alternative approaches to health care ethics but has decided to include a discussion of what is referred to as 'the ethics of care' in the third section of her assignment. For this activity, provide a brief account of the key features of the ethics of care and how it can be understood as highlighting the potential limitations of principlism as an approach to health care ethics.

An outline answer is provided at the end of the chapter.

Concluding the work

Having provided an introduction to your critical writing and, in accordance with the rule of three, structured that work into three equal sections that are characterised by a systematic, coherent and logical progression, it is necessary to provide a conclusion to your work. In doing so, it is important to recognise that your conclusion ought to be a brief summary of what you have discussed in your critical writing and which highlights the main points, issues or claims that you have explored over the course of your critical discussion. The conclusion is therefore not the place to introduce new concepts, to develop new arguments or to consider critically the complexity of the area of mental health care under investigation; rather, any points, issues or claims that you wish to explore ought to be incorporated into one of the three sections that characterises the rule of three. In order to ensure that your conclusion does not introduce new material that would require further elaboration and critical discussion, it can be productive to understand that conclusion in terms of a 'mirror image', or as possessing the same essential structure, as your introduction. That is, while your introduction is a brief outline of what you intend to discuss in the first, second and third section of your critical writing, your conclusion can be understood as providing a similarly brief summary of what you have discussed in those respective sections and, importantly, how you have conducted that discussion. In this way, you contribute to the sense that your critical writing is an integrated, coherent and progressive whole in which your introduction provides an account of what you are going to do in your critical writing; then, in each of the sections that comprise the rule of three, you engage in what you had proposed to do and, finally, you conclude your critical writing by confirming what it is that you have done.

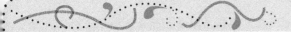

Chapter summary

This chapter has discussed the importance of critical writing and being able to develop the ability to engage in that form of writing for your university assignments. In doing so, it has examined in detail what is referred to as the rule of three, which is a way of understanding your critical writing, and indeed any other form of writing that you may conduct during your mental health nursing programme, in terms of an equally distributed and developmental three-part structure that can help you to organise and express the content of your work in a systematic, coherent and convincing manner. In particular, we have examined how the first section of that three-part structure requires you to establish what the area or issue under investigation is going to be, to set the scene or lay the foundations for what you are going to discuss critically; we have also examined the manner in which the second section of that three-part structure requires you to develop the central features of the area of mental health care under investigation, to move the discussion along, and do so by adding further detail, depth and breadth of thought to your critical writing; finally, we have also examined the manner in which the third section of the three-part structure that characterises the rule of three requires you, as it were, to arrive somewhere, to bring the varied elements of your investigation together in such a way that you are able to reach some form of conclusion, however provisional or tentative it may be. As with all of the skills and attributes associated with critical thinking and reflection, the ability to produce coherent and convincing critical writing will take time, practice and patience to develop; however, this chapter has encouraged you to begin to think about, and strive to work in accordance with, the rule of three in order to begin to develop your ability to produce consistently high-quality critical writing for your mental health nursing programme.

Activities: brief outline answers

Activity 9.1 Decision making

When considering how to divide Ruth's 2,000-word essay numerically into an overarching three-part structure that gives equal consideration to each of those three sections, you may have identified various alternative forms. However, one of the most straightforward would be to allocate 250 words for a more substantial introduction to her critical discussion and 250 words for a similarly substantial conclusion. Doing so would leave Ruth with 1,500 words which, using the rule of three, could be divided into three sections of 500 words while each section could, in turn, be further divided into two paragraphs of 250 words.

Activity 9.2 Evidence-based practice and research

In accessing the Care Quality Commission's (2015) most recent annual report into the use of the Mental Health Act 1983, you may have discovered many significant features about the contemporary use of compulsory powers under the Act, including, for example, the continued higher rates of people from black and minority ethnic communities being detained. However, when considering what information to include in the introduction to Ruth's critical writing, you might have discovered that there were 23,531 people subject to the Act in 2013–2014: 18,166 of those people were detained in hospital and 5,365 people were subject to a community treatment order; this represents a 6 per cent increase in the number of people subject to the Act when compared with the 2012–2013 reporting year and a 32 per cent increase since 2008–2009, which was the reporting year in which community treatment orders were introduced (Health & Social Care Information Centre 2014; Care Quality Commission 2015).

Activity 9.3 Critical thinking

In demonstrating your knowledge and comprehension of the notion of paternalism by situating it in a clinical context you may have identified numerous clinical examples of acts, practices or policies in contemporary mental health care that could be considered paternalistic. For example, any form of compulsory treatment, the use of physical restraint and seclusion, the employment of 'close' or 'special' observations and the covert administration of medication can all be understood as explicit instances of paternalism. However, it has been suggested that a variety of less 'formal' instances of paternalism exist in contemporary mental health care including, for example, the rationing of a person's cigarettes, the imposition of what, when and where people eat and the withholding and manipulation of information about the adverse effects of psychiatric medication (Roberts 2004; Lakeman 2009).

Activity 9.4 Team working

In considering the argument that the use of compulsory powers under the Mental Health Act 1983 is justified with reference to beneficence and non-maleficence, that such powers ensure good and prevent harm, you may have had informative, complex and stimulating conversations with your colleagues. For example, you may have had a thought-provoking discussion about what constitutes 'good' and 'harm' and from whose perspective such judgements are to be made: from the perspective of those who use mental health services, from the perspective of mental health professionals or from the perspective of society more generally. You may also have had interesting discussions about the significance of the notion of 'mental disorder' or 'mental illness' when considering the ethical justification for the use of compulsory powers under the Mental Health Act 1983. Indeed, acts of paternalism in contemporary mental health care, such as the use of compulsory powers, are often not only justified by suggesting that they ensure good and prevent harm, but also by proposing that the person who is subject to such acts has a mental disorder and, as a consequence, has a diminished capacity to act in an autonomous manner and determine what is in his or her best interests (Beauchamp & Childress 2001; Roberts 2004). However, you may have had detailed discussions about what constitutes capacity, the means by which a person's capacity can be assessed and the extent to which mental disorder can be understood as diminishing a person's capacity to act in an autonomous manner. Finally, you may have informed your discussion with reference to various forms of ethical, professional and legal documentation associated with the use of compulsory powers under the Mental Health Act 1983, including the Code of Practice (DH 2015a), the Human Rights Act 1998 and the Mental Capacity Act 2005.

Activity 9.5 Evidence-based practice and research

Building upon the work of a number of feminist writers, including Carol Gilligan (1982) and Nel Noddings (1984), the ethics of care stresses the importance of attending to particular situations, contexts and relationships when attempting to understand and respond to ethical issues in contemporary health care. In contrast to principlism, and its employment of general principles such as autonomy, beneficence and non-maleficence, the ethics of care emphasises the need for an 'engaged involvement' with ethical issues and, in order to achieve this, the importance of emotional responsiveness within health care relationships (Allmark 1995). In doing so, principlism is presented as a form of rational, universal and detached ethical reasoning that is said to be inappropriate in the context of contemporary health care, and particularly in contemporary mental health care, in which there is an emphasis on developing therapeutic relationships and supportive alliances with those who use health care services. In contrast to the priority that principlism is said to give to rational, universal and detached ethical reasoning, the ethics of care stresses the importance of both reason and emotion when attempting to understand and respond to ethical issues, to recognise that appropriate ethical decision making occurs within the context of unique interpersonal relationships and the particular health care situation in which both service users and health care professionals are positioned.

Further reading

Cottrell S (2011) *Critical Thinking Skills: Developing effective analysis and argument*, 2nd edition. Basingstoke: Palgrave Macmillan.

Although not specific to health care, this book provides a comprehensive account of how to develop a range of critical thinking skills, including how to identify, evaluate and develop arguments and how to incorporate these into your critical, analytical writing.

Gimenez J (2011) *Writing for Nursing and Midwifery Students*, 2nd edition. Basingstoke: Palgrave Macmillan.

This is a comprehensive introduction to the various forms of academic writing that nursing students are required to engage in over the course of their studies and also includes detailed guidance on how to write an argument.

Peck J & Coyle M (2012) *The Student's Guide to Writing: Spelling, punctuation and grammar*, 3rd edition. Basingstoke: Palgrave Macmillan.

A highly accessible and informative introduction to writing for students that includes, among other things, an extended discussion about how to write systematic, coherent and convincing essays using the rule of three.

Price B & Harrington A (2013) *Critical Thinking and Writing for Nursing Students*, 2nd edition. London: Sage/Learning Matters.

This book provides an accessible introduction to critical thinking and writing for nursing students and includes practical instruction on how to develop the skills and attributes necessary for writing critical, analytical essays.

Useful websites

www.rlf.org.uk/resource/writing-essays

Here you will find an accessible, detailed and practical resource from the Royal Literary Fund on how to write essays at a university level that guides you, in a systematic manner, through each stage of the essay-writing process.

Glossary

Accountability: the condition of being answerable and responsible for one's actions and decisions.

Acculturation: the process of change that occurs when an individual or group from one culture encounters an individual or group from other cultures.

Aesthetic: relating to art, beauty and creativity.

Affective: relating to moods, feelings and attitudes.

Anthropological: relating to the study of humankind, and especially the origins and development of past and present cultures and societies.

Autocratic: relating to autocracy and the political principle that the decisions that affect a group of people should be made by one person.

Autonomy: the right, condition or capacity to make decisions and act in a manner that is free from undue control, constraint and influence.

Beneficence: the principle and practice of acting in a way that seeks to benefit others and ensure good.

Cognitive: relating to intellectual activity, such as analysing, reasoning and remembering.

Consumerism: the principle and practice of pursuing and obtaining material goods, products and services.

Core conditions: in the context of person-centred therapy and interpersonal communication more generally, the conditions or qualities that are considered necessary to establish therapeutic relationships and bring about therapeutic change (i.e. empathy, genuineness and unconditional positive regard).

Critical evaluation: the practice of systematically thinking about a piece of information in order to determine its worth and importance.

Democratic: relating to democracy and the political principle that the decisions that affect a group of people should be made by those people.

Discrimination: the practice of treating a person or people less favourably because they possess, or are perceived as possessing, a particular characteristic.

Disease-centred model: in the context of medication, the explanation that psychiatric drugs work by targeting specific underlying disease processes.

Drug-centred model: in contrast to the disease-centred model, the explanation that psychiatric drugs produce a range of altered mental and physical states that may have both a negative and positive effect on the person and the symptoms associated with mental distress.

Egocentrism: the condition of thinking, feeling and acting from one's own perspective without giving due consideration to alternative perspectives.

Embodying: the practice of giving concrete form and expression to an idea, quality or disposition.

Empirical: relating to observation, experience and experiment.

Ethics: standards of right and wrong conduct and also a branch of philosophy that is concerned with questioning, analysing and reasoning about what is right and wrong conduct.

Evidence-based practice: the explicit use of the best current evidence when considering which interventions and treatments to provide to those who use health care services.

Existential problems: relating to questions, issues and problems surrounding human existence, particularly the purpose, direction and meaning of one's life.

Homogeneous: the quality of being similar or the same.

Individualism: a belief in the worth of the individual and the right of each individual to decide and pursue what is in his or her best interests.

Institutional racism: the perpetuation of negative attitudes and unequal treatment by an institution towards a person or people based on their race.

Leading by example: the practice of consistently acting in a way that sets a desirable standard for others to emulate and follow.

Liberalism: the political principle and practice of protecting and enhancing the rights, freedom and liberty of the individual.

Managerialism: the principle and practice of using professional managers to plan and administer the activities of a group of individuals. It is associated with the importance of setting targets, and obtaining those targets with maximum efficiency.

Mass media: relating to the forms of communication that are designed to reach large numbers of people, such as television, films and newspapers.

Modelling: the practice of performing certain competencies in such a way that one's actions can serve as an example, standard or model from which others can learn. It can also refer to the practice of learning from others by observing the manner in which they perform certain competencies.

Non-attachment: the condition or practice of relating to events, and one's thoughts and feelings about those events, in a calm, composed and balanced manner.

Non-maleficence: the principle and practice of acting in a way that does not harm others.

Norms: beliefs, attitudes and behaviors that are considered normal in a particular group, culture or society.

Open questions: questions which cannot be answered with 'yes' or 'no' and therefore enable a person to 'open up' and respond to a question in detail.

Paradigm: a collection of assumptions, concepts and theories that form a framework by which to understand an aspect of the world or the world more generally.

Paraphrasing: the practice of restating something that has been written or spoken using different words.

Paternalism: the principle and practice of limiting, obstructing or overriding the freedom, self-determination and autonomy of others.

Peer-reviewed: relating to the evaluation of a person's work by others who work in that area and possess a similar level of expertise.

Plagiarism: the practice of using someone else's words, thoughts and ideas and, intentionally or unintentionally, presenting them as your own.

Polypharmacy: the practice of prescribing 'multiple' medications (commonly understood as four or more) to the same individual.

Prejudice: a preconceived and often negative opinion about others that is formed without good reason.

Qualitative research methodologies: research frameworks or approaches – such as phenomenology, grounded theory, ethnography and case studies – that are adopted to carry out research into people's experiences and the quality of those experiences.

Quantitative research methodologies: research frameworks or approaches – such as randomised controlled trials, cohort studies, case-control studies and cross-sectional studies – that are adopted to obtain measurable or quantifiable data.

Randomised controlled trial: a research experiment in which participants are randomly assigned to receive one of two or more treatment interventions to determine the usefulness of those interventions.

Reflection-in-action: the process by which a person thinks about his or her activity while in the midst of it.

Reflection-on-action: the process by which a person thinks about his or her activity after it has finished.

Self-determination: the right, condition or capacity to decide what is in one's best interests and act in a manner that is free from undue control, constraint and influence.

Sick role: relating to the set of beliefs, behaviours and expectations associated with being sick that are placed upon someone or that an individual may adopt.

Signs: in the context of health care, the physical indications of the potential presence of disease or disorder.

Social determinants: the social and economic conditions that affect, influence and determine the health of individuals.

Stereotypical: relating to a fixed and oversimplified image or idea about an individual or a group.

Stigma: a characteristic that is judged to be unwanted and shameful and the disapproval of a person because he or she possesses, or is perceived as possessing, this characteristic.

Symptoms: the subjective experiences and feelings about the potential presence of disease or disorder that a person may report to health care professionals.

Technocratic: relating to technocracy and the political principle that the decisions that affect a group of people should be made by individuals who possess technical knowledge and expertise.

Values-based practice: the practice of recognising and working with one's personal values, professional values and the values of those who use health care services when considering which interventions and treatments to provide.

References

Adams T & Collier E (2009) Services for older people with mental health conditions, in Barker P (ed) *Psychiatric and Mental Health Nursing: The craft of caring*, 2nd edition. London: Hodder Arnold, pp. 486–92.

Allmark P (1995) Can there be an ethics of care? *Journal of Medical Ethics*, 21(1): 19–24.

Anderson D (2011) Age discrimination in mental health services needs to be understood. *The Psychiatrist*, 35(1): 1–4.

Anthony WA (1993) Recovery from mental illness: the guiding vision of the mental health system in the 1990s. *Psychosocial Rehabilitation Journal*, 16(4): 11–23.

APA (American Psychiatric Association) (2013) *Diagnostic and Statistical Manual of Mental Disorders*, 5th edition (DSM-5). Washington, DC: American Psychiatric Association.

Arpa M (2013) *Mindfulness at Work: Flourishing in the workplace*. Lewes: Leaping Hare Press.

Aveyard H, Sharp P & Woolliams M (2015) *A Beginner's Guide to Critical Thinking and Writing in Health and Social Care*, 2nd edition. Maidenhead: Open University Press.

Barber P, Brown R & Martin D (2012) *Mental Health Law in England and Wales: A guide for mental health professionals*, 2nd edition. London: Sage/Learning Matters.

Barker P (2009a) The nature of nursing, in Barker P (ed) *Psychiatric and Mental Health Nursing: The craft of caring*, 2nd edition. London: Hodder Arnold, pp. 3–11.

Barker P (2009b) Psychiatric nursing, in Barker P (ed) *Psychiatric and Mental Health Nursing: The craft of caring*, 2nd edition. London: Hodder Arnold, pp 123–32.

Barker P & Buchanan-Barker P (2009) Getting personal: being human in mental health care, in Barker P (ed) *Psychiatric and Mental Health Nursing: The craft of caring*, 2nd edition. London: Hodder Arnold, pp. 12–20.

Basaglia F (1981) Breaking the circuit of control, in Ingleby D (ed) *Critical Psychiatry: The politics of mental health*. Harmondsworth: Penguin, pp. 184–92.

Beauchamp TL (2000) The philosophical basis of psychiatric ethics, in Bloch S & Green SA (eds) *Psychiatric Ethics*, 4th edition. New York: Oxford University Press, pp. 25–48.

Beauchamp TL & Childress JF (2001) *Principles of Biomedical Ethics*, 5th edition. New York: Oxford University Press.

Beck AT, Rush AJ, Shaw BF & Emery G (1979) *Cognitive Therapy of Depression*. New York: The Guilford Press.

Beecham J, Knapp M, Fernández JL, Huxley P, Mangalore R, McCrone P, Snell T, Winter B & Wittenberg R (2008) *Age Discrimination in Mental Health Services*. Canterbury: PSSRU.

Ben-Zeev D, Young MA & Corrigan PW (2010) DSM-V and the stigma of mental illness. *Journal of Mental Health*, 19(4): 318–27.

Bentall RP (2004) *Madness Explained: Psychosis and human nature*. London: Penguin.

Bentall RP (2010) *Doctoring the Mind: Why psychiatric treatments fail*. London: Penguin.

Beresford P (2010) *A Straight Talking Introduction to Being a Mental Health Service User*. Ross-on-Wye: PCCS Books.

Beresford P (2013) *Beyond the Usual Suspects: Towards inclusive user involvement*. London: Shaping Our Lives.

Biggs S, Phillipson C, Leach R & Money A (2007) Baby boomers and adult ageing: issues for social and public policy. *Quality in Ageing and Older Adults*, 8(3): 32–40.

Boardman J & Roberts G (2014) *Risk, Safety and Recovery*. London: Centre for Mental Health and Mental Health Network, NHS Confederation.

Bolton G (2014) *Reflective Practice: Writing and professional development*, 4th edition. London: Sage.

Borton T (1970) *Reach, Touch and Teach*. New York: McGraw-Hill.

Boud D, Keogh R & Walker D (1985) Promoting reflection in learning: a model, in Boud D, Keogh R & Walker D (eds) *Reflection: Turning experience into learning.* London: Kogan Page, pp. 18–40.

Bourdieu P (1992) *Language and Symbolic Power.* Cambridge: Polity Press.

Boyd EM & Fayles AW (1983) Reflective learning: key to learning from experience. *Journal of Humanistic Psychology,* 23(2): 99–117.

Boyle M (2002) *Schizophrenia: A scientific delusion,* 2nd edition. London: Routledge.

Boyle M (2012) Diagnosis, in Newness C, Holmes G & Dunn C (eds) *This is Madness: A critical look at psychiatry and the future of mental health services.* Ross-on-Wye: PCCS Books, pp. 75–90.

Bracken P & Thomas P (2001) Postpsychiatry: a new direction for mental health. *British Medical Journal,* 322: 724–7.

Breggin P (1993) *Toxic Psychiatry.* London: Fontana.

Brookfield SD (2001) *Developing Critical Thinkers: Challenging adults to explore alternative ways of thinking and acting.* Milton Keynes: Open University Press.

Bulman C & Schutz S (eds) (2013) *Reflective Practice in Nursing,* 5th edition. Chichester: John Wiley.

Busfield J (2011) *Mental Illness.* Cambridge: Polity Press.

Cahill J, Paley G & Hardy G (2013) What do patients find helpful in psychotherapy? Implications for the therapeutic relationship in mental health nursing. *Journal of Psychiatric and Mental Health Nursing,* 20(9): 782–91.

Campbell P (2013) Service users/survivors and mental health services, in Cromby J, Harper D & Reavey P (eds) *Psychology, Mental Health and Distress.* Basingstoke: Palgrave Macmillan, pp. 139–51.

Care Quality Commission (2015) *Monitoring the Mental Health Act in 2013/14.* London: HMSO.

Carper BA (1978) Fundamental patterns of knowing in nursing. *Advances in Nursing Science,* 1(1): 13–23.

Castillo H (2003) *Personality Disorder: Temperament or trauma?* London: Jessica Kingsley.

Chamberlin J (1977) *On Our Own.* London: Mind.

Chesler P (1972) *Women and Madness.* New York: Doubleday.

Coleman R (1999) *Recovery: An alien concept.* Gloucester: Handsell Publishing.

Cooper D (1967) *Psychiatry and Anti-Psychiatry.* London: Tavistock Publications.

Cooper M (2008) *Essential Research Findings in Counselling and Psychotherapy.* London: Sage.

Cooper M & McLeod J (2011) *Pluralistic Counselling and Psychotherapy.* London: Sage.

Coppock V (2008) Gender, in Tummey R & Turner T (eds) *Critical Issues in Mental Health.* Basingstoke: Palgrave Macmillan, pp. 91–107.

Copus J (2009) *Brilliant Writing Tips for Students.* Basingstoke: Palgrave Macmillan.

Cottrell S (2011) *Critical Thinking Skills: Developing effective analysis and argument,* 2nd edition. Basingstoke: Palgrave Macmillan.

Courtenay WH (2000) Constructions of masculinity and their influence on men's well-being: a theory of gender and health. *Social Science and Medicine,* 50: 1385–1401.

Cromby J, Harper D & Reavey P (2013a) Disordered personalities? in Cromby J, Harper D & Reavey P (eds) *Psychology, Mental Health and Distress.* Basingstoke: Palgrave Macmillan, pp. 308–38.

Cromby J, Harper D & Reavey P (2013b) From disorder to experience, in Cromby J, Harper D & Reavey P (eds) *Psychology, Mental Health and Distress.* Basingstoke: Palgrave Macmillan, pp. 3–18.

Crowe M & Carlyle D (2009) The person with a diagnosis of personality disorder, in Barker P (ed) *Psychiatric and Mental Health Nursing: The craft of caring,* 2nd edition. London: Hodder Arnold, pp. 244–51.

Curtis T, Dellar R, Leslie E & Watson B (eds) (2000) *Mad Pride: A celebration of mad culture.* London: Spare Change Books.

Cutcliffe J & Santos JC (2012) *Suicide and Self-Harm: An evidence-informed approach.* London: Quay Books.

de Beauvoir S (2015/1949) *The Second Sex.* London: Vintage.

Deegan P (1988) Recovery: the lived experience of rehabilitation. *Psychosocial Rehabilitation Journal,* 11(4): 11–19.

Deleuze G & Guattari F (2000/1972) *Anti-Oedipus: Capitalism and schizophrenia.* London: Athlone.

Dewar B, Adamson E, Smith S, Surfleet J & King L (2014) Clarifying misconceptions about compassionate care. *Journal of Advanced Nursing,* 70(8): 1738–47.

Dewey J (1997/1938) *Experience and Education.* New York: Simon & Schuster.

Dewey J (2012/1910) *How We Think.* Mansfield Centre, CT: Martino Publishing.

DH (Department of Health) (2004) *The Ten Essential Shared Capabilities: A framework for the whole of the mental health workforce.* London: Department of Health.

DH (Department of Health) (2006) *From Values to Action: The Chief Nursing Officer's review of mental health nursing.* London: Department of Health.

DH (Department of Health) (2009) *Living Well With Dementia: A national dementia strategy.* London: Department of Health.

DH (Department of Health) (2011a) *No Health Without Mental Health: A cross-government mental health outcomes strategy for people of all ages.* London: Department of Health.

DH (Department of Health) (2011b) *Talking Therapies: A four year plan of action.* London: Department of Health.

DH (Department of Health) (2012) *Compassion in Practice: Nursing, midwifery and care staff – our vision and strategy.* London: Department of Health.

DH (Department of Health) (2014) *Closing the Gap: Priorities for essential change in mental health.* London: Department of Health.

DH (Department of Health) (2015a) *Mental Health Act 1983: Code of practice.* London: The Stationery Office.

DH (Department of Health) (2015b) *Reference Guide to the Mental Health Act 1983.* London: The Stationery Office.

Doherty DT & Kartalova-O'Doherty Y (2010) Gender and self-reported mental health problems: predictors of help seeking from a general practitioner. *The British Journal of Health Psychology,* 15: 213–28.

Egan G (2014) *The Skilled Helper: A problem-management and opportunity-development approach to helping,* 10th edition. Belmont, CA: Brooks/Cole, Cengage Learning.

Elliot L & Masters H (2009) Mental health inequalities and mental health nursing. *Journal of Psychiatric and Mental Health Nursing,* 16(8): 762–71.

Ellis A (1962) *Reason and Emotion in Psychotherapy.* New York: Lyle Stuart.

Fairclough N (2015) *Language and Power,* 3rd edition. London: Routledge.

Fanon F (2001/1961) *The Wretched of the Earth.* London: Penguin.

Faulkner A & Thomas P (2002) User-led research and evidence-based medicine. *British Journal of Psychiatry,* 180(1): 1–3.

Fernando S (2008) Institutional racism and cultural diversity, in Tummey R & Turner T (eds) *Critical Issues in Mental Health.* Basingstoke: Palgrave Macmillan, pp. 41–57.

Fernando S (2010) *Mental Health, Race and Culture,* 3rd edition. Basingstoke: Palgrave Macmillan.

Foucault M (2001/1961) *Madness and Civilization: A history of insanity in the age of reason.* London: Routledge.

Foucault M (2005/1966) *The Order of Things: An archaeology of the human sciences.* London: Routledge.

Fulford KWM (2007) Facts/values: Ten principles of values-based medicine, in Radden J (ed) *The Philosophy of Psychiatry: A companion.* New York: Oxford University Press, pp. 205–34.

Fulford KWM (2008) Values-based practice: a new partner to evidence-based practice and a first for psychiatry? *Mens Sana Monograhs,* 6(1): 10–21.

Fulford KWM, Peile E & Carroll H (2012) *Essential Values-Based Practice: Clinical stories linking science with people.* New York: Cambridge University Press.

Furedi F (2004) *Therapy Culture: Cultivating vulnerability in an uncertain age.* London: Routledge.

Geddes JR & Harrison PJ (1997) Closing the gap between research and practice. *British Journal of Psychiatry,* 171: 220–5.

Gibbs G (1988) *Learning by Doing: A guide to teaching and learning methods.* Oxford: Further Education Unit, Oxford Polytechnic.

Gilligan C (1982) *In a Different Voice: Psychological theory and women's development.* Cambridge, MA: Harvard University Press.

Gimenez J (2011) *Writing for Nursing and Midwifery Students,* 2nd edition. Basingstoke: Palgrave Macmillan.

Goffman E (1961) *Asylums: Essays on the social situation of mental patients and other inmates.* New York: Doubleday Anchor.

Goffman E (1963) *Stigma: Notes on the management of a spoiled identity.* Englewood Cliffs, NJ: Prentice-Hall.

Greenhalgh T (2014) *How to Read a Paper: The basics of evidence-based medicine,* 5th edition. Chichester: John Wiley.

Gunn JS & Potter B (2015) *Borderline Personality Disorder: New perspectives on a stigmatizing and overused diagnosis.* Santa Barbara: Praeger.

Guyatt GH, Sackett DL, Sinclair JC, Hayward R, Cook DJ & Cook RJ (1995) Users' guide to the medical literature: IX. A method for grading health care recommendations. *Journal of the American Medical Association,* 274(22): 1800–4.

Gøtzsche PC (2013) *Deadly Medicines and Organised Crime: How big pharma has corrupted healthcare.* London: Radcliffe Publishing.

Hare RM (1952) *The Language of Morals.* Oxford: Oxford University Press.

Health Committee (2014) *Children's and adolescents' mental health and CAMHS.* London: The Stationery Office.

Health & Social Care Information Centre (2014) *Inpatients Formally Detained in Hospitals Under the Mental Health Act 1983, and Patients Subject to Supervised Community Treatment: Annual report, England, 2013/14.* London: Health & Social Care Information Centre.

Heath M (2012) On critical thinking. *The International Journal of Narrative Therapy and Community Work,* 4: 11–18.

Henderson L (2008) Media: reframing the debates, in Tummey R & Turner T (eds) *Critical Issues in Mental Health.* Basingstoke: Palgrave Macmillan, pp. 195–212.

Hinshaw SP (2010) *The Mark of Shame: Stigma of mental illness and an agenda for change.* New York: Oxford University Press.

Hitchen S, Watkins M, Williamson GR, Ambury S, Bemrose G, Cook D & Taylor M (2011) Lone voices have an emotional content: focussing on mental health service user and carer involvement. *International Journal of Health Care Quality Assurance,* 24(2): 164–77.

Holland K & Hogg C (2010) *Cultural Awareness in Nursing and Health Care: An introductory text,* 2nd edition. Boca Raton, FL: CRC Press.

Honos-Webb L & Leitner LM (2001) How using the DSM causes damage: a client's report. *Journal of Humanistic Psychology,* 41(4): 36–56.

Howatson-Jones L (2013) *Reflective Practice in Nursing,* 2nd edition. London: Sage/Learning Matters.

Ingleby D (1981) Understanding 'mental illness', in Ingleby D (ed) *Critical Psychiatry: The politics of mental health.* Harmondsworth: Penguin, pp. 23–71.

Ion RM & Beer MD (2002) The British reaction to dementia praecox 1893–1913. Part 1. *History of Psychiatry,* 13: 285–304.

Jasper M (2003) *Foundations in Nursing and Health Care: Beginning reflective practice.* Cheltenham: Nelson Thornes.

Jasper M (2006) Reflection and reflective practice, in Jasper M (ed) *Professional Development, Reflection and Decision-Making.* Oxford: Blackwell Publishing, pp. 39–80.

JCPMH (Joint Commissioning Panel for Mental Health) (2014) *Guidance for Commissioners of Mental Health Services for People from Black and Minority Ethnic Communities.* London: JCPMH.

Johns C (2004) *Becoming a Reflective Practitioner*, 2nd edition. Oxford: Blackwell Publishing.

Johnstone L (2000) *Users and Abusers of Psychiatry: A critical look at psychiatric practice*, 2nd edition. London: Routledge.

Johnstone L (2008) Psychiatric diagnosis, in Tummey R & Turner T (eds) *Critical Issues in Mental Health*. Basingstoke: Palgrave Macmillan, pp. 5–22.

Johnstone L (2013) Diagnosis and formulation, in Cromby J, Harper D & Reavey P (eds) *Psychology, Mental Health and Distress*. Basingstoke: Palgrave Macmillan, pp. 101–17.

Johnstone L (2014) *A Straight Talking Introduction to Psychiatric Diagnosis*. Ross-on-Wye: PCCS Books.

Kelly P & Moloney P (2013) Psychological therapies, in Cromby J, Harper D & Reavey P (eds) *Psychology, Mental Health and Distress*. Basingstoke: Palgrave Macmillan, pp. 173–9.

Kim HS (1999) Critical reflective inquiry for knowledge development in nursing practice. *Journal of Advance Nursing*, 29(5): 1205–12.

Kolb DA (1984) *Experiential Learning: Experience as the source of learning and development*. Englewood Cliffs, NJ: Prentice Hall.

Laing RD (1960) *The Divided Self*. London: Tavistock Publications.

Lakeman R (2009) Ethics and nursing, in Barker P (ed) *Psychiatric and Mental Health Nursing: The craft of caring*, 2nd edition. London: Hodder Arnold, pp. 607–17.

Lauder W, Kroll T & Jones M (2007) Social determinants of mental health: the missing dimensions of mental health nursing? *Journal of Psychiatric and Mental Health Nursing*, 14(7): 661–9.

LeFrançois BA, Menzies R & Reaume G (eds) (2013) *Mad Matters: A critical reader in Canadian mad studies*. Toronto: Canadian Scholars' Press.

Link BG & Phelan JC (2001) Conceptualizing stigma. *Annual Review of Sociology*, 27: 363–85.

Littlewood R & Lipsedge M (1997) *Aliens and Alienists: Ethnic minorities and psychiatry*, 3rd edition. London: Routledge.

Luborsky L, Rosenthal R, Diguer L, Andrusyna TP, Berman JS, Levitt JT, Seligman DA & Krause ED (2002) The dodo bird verdict is alive and well – mostly. *Clinical Psychology: Science and Practice*, 9(1): 2–12.

Maccallum EJ (2002) Othering and psychiatric nursing. *Journal of Psychiatric and Mental Health Nursing*, 9(1): 87–96.

Macpherson W (1999) *The Stephen Lawrence Inquiry: Report of an inquiry by Sir William Macpherson of Cluny*. London: The Stationery Office.

Maltby J, Williams G, McGarry J & Day L (2010) *Research Methods for Nursing and Healthcare*. Harlow: Pearson Education.

Mantzoukas S (2008) A review of evidence-based practice, nursing research and reflection: levelling the hierarchy. *Journal of Clinical Nursing*, 17(2): 214–23.

Masson J (1988) *Against Therapy: Emotional tyranny and the myth of psychological healing*. New York: Atheneum.

McKenna H (2009) Evidence-based practice in mental health, in Barker P (ed) *Psychiatric and Mental Health Nursing: The craft of caring*, 2nd edition. London: Hodder Arnold, pp. 30–6.

McKenzie K & Bhui K (2007) Institutional racism in mental health care. *British Medical Journal*, 334: 649–50.

McLean C, Fulford B & Carpenter D (2012) Values-based practice, in Tee S, Brown J & Carpenter D (eds) *Handbook of Mental Health Nursing*. London: Hodder Arnold, pp. 55–72.

Mental Health Foundation (2009) *All Things Being Equal: Age equality in mental health care for older people in England*. London: Mental Health Foundation.

Mezirow J (1991) *Transformative Dimensions of Adult Learning*. San Francisco: Jossey-Bass.

Miller J (2013) *The Philosophical Life: Twelve great thinkers and the search for wisdom, from Socrates to Nietzsche*. London: Oneworld Publications.

Moloney P (2013) *The Therapy Industry: The irresistible rise of the talking cure, and why it doesn't work*. London: Pluto Press.

Moncrieff J (2008) *The Myth of the Chemical Cure: A critique of psychiatric drug treatment.* Basingstoke: Palgrave Macmillan.

Moncrieff J (2013) Psychiatric medication, in Cromby J, Harper D & Reavey P (eds) *Psychology, Mental Health and Distress.* Basingstoke: Palgrave Macmillan, pp. 160–8.

Moncrieff J & Cohen D (2009) How do psychiatric drugs work? *British Medical Journal,* 338: 1535–7.

Moncrieff J, Cohen D & Porter S (2013) The psychoactive effects of psychiatric medication: the elephant in the room. *Journal of Psychoactive Drugs,* 45(5): 409–15.

Morgan G (2006) *Images of Organization,* 4th edition. Thousand Oaks, CA: Sage.

Morgan S (2013) *Risk Decision-Making: Working with risk and implementing positive risk-taking.* Hove: Pavilion.

Moule P & Goodman M (2014) *Nursing Research: An introduction,* 2nd edition. London: Sage.

Murphy R & Wales P (2013) *Mental Health Law in Nursing.* London: Sage/Learning Matters.

NIMHE (National Institute for Mental Health in England) (2003) *Inside Outside: Improving mental health services for black and minority ethnic communities in England.* Leeds: NIMHE.

NMC (Nursing & Midwifery Council) (2010) *Standards for Pre-registration Nursing Education.* London: NMC.

NMC (Nursing & Midwifery Council) (2015) *The Code: Professional standards of practice and behaviour for nurses and midwifes.* London: NMC.

Noddings N (1984) *Caring: A feminine approach to ethics and moral education.* Berkeley, CA: University of California Press.

Norcross JC (ed) (2011) *Psychotherapy Relationships That Work: Evidence-based responsiveness,* 2nd edition. New York: Oxford University Press.

Norfolk, Suffolk & Cambridgeshire Strategic Health Authority (2003) *Independent Inquiry into the Death of David Bennett.* Cambridge: Norfolk, Suffolk & Cambridgeshire Strategic Health Authority.

NSUN (National Service User Network) (2015a) *Involvement for Influence: The 4Pi standards for involvement.* London: NSUN.

NSUN (National Service User Network) (2015b) *The Language of Mental Wellbeing.* London: NSUN.

O'Brien AJ, Morrison E & DeSouza R (2009) Providing culturally safe care, in Barker P (ed) *Psychiatric and Mental Health Nursing: The craft of caring,* 2nd edition. London: Hodder Arnold, pp. 635–43.

O'Halloran P, Porter S & Blackwood B (2010) Evidence based practice and its critics: what is a nurse manager to do? *Journal of Nursing Management,* 18(1): 90–5.

Osmond A (2013) *Academic Writing and Grammar for Students.* London: Sage.

Patel K & Heginbotham C (2007) Institutional racism in mental health services does not imply racism in individual psychiatrists: commentary on . . . Institutional racism in psychiatry. *Psychiatric Bulletin,* 31: 367–8.

Paul R & Elder L (2014) *Critical Thinking: Tools for taking charge of your professional and personal life,* 2nd edition. Upper Saddle River, NJ: Pearson Education.

Peck J & Coyle M (2012) *The Student's Guide to Writing: Spelling, punctuation and grammar,* 3rd edition. Basingstoke: Palgrave Macmillan.

Pelle J (2014) Cross-cultural communication, in Walker S (ed) *Engagement and Therapeutic Communication in Mental Health Nursing.* London: Sage/Learning Matters, pp. 98–112.

Philo G, Henderson L & McCracken K (2010) *Making Drama Out of a Crisis: Authentic portrayals of mental illness in TV drama.* London: Shift.

Piaget J (1959) *The Language and Thought of the Child.* London: Routledge & Kegan Paul.

Pilgrim D (2007) The survival of psychiatric diagnosis. *Social Science & Medicine,* 65: 536–47.

Pilgrim D & McCranie A (2013) *Recovery and Mental Health: A critical sociological account.* Basingstoke: Palgrave Macmillan.

Plato (1961) The apology, in Hamilton E & Cairns H (eds) *The Collected Dialogues of Plato.* Princeton: Princeton University Press, pp. 3–26.

Porter R (2003) *Madness: A brief history.* Oxford: Oxford University Press.

Potter N (2007) Gender, in Radden J (ed) *The Philosophy of Psychiatry: A companion*. New York: Oxford University Press, pp. 237–43.

Price B & Harrington A (2013) *Critical Thinking and Writing for Nursing Students*, 2nd edition. London: Sage/Learning Matters.

Proctor G (2007) Disordered boundaries? A critique of 'borderline personality disorder', in Spandler H & Warner S (eds) *Beyond Fear and Control: Working with young people who self-harm*. Ross-on-Wye: PCCS Books, pp. 105–18.

Rayner L (2014) Stress vulnerability and psychosis, in Stickley T & Wright N (eds) *Theories for Mental Health Nursing: A guide for practice*. London: Sage, pp. 202–22.

Reeves A (2010) *Counselling Suicidal Clients*. London: Sage.

Repper J & Perkins R (2003) *Social Inclusion and Recovery: A model for mental health practice*. London: Baillière Tindall.

Repper J & Perkins R (2014) Why recovery? in Stickley T & Wright N (eds) *Theories for Mental Health Nursing: A guide for practice*. London: Sage, pp. 183–201.

Roberts G & Boardman J (2014) Becoming a recovery-oriented practitioner. *Advances in Psychiatric Treatment*, 20(1): 37–47.

Roberts J (2015) Mindfulness for all in action, in Walker S (ed) *Psychosocial Interventions in Mental Health Nursing*. London: Sage/Learning Matters, pp. 63–80.

Roberts M (2004) Psychiatric ethics: a critical introduction for mental health nurses. *Journal of Psychiatric and Mental Health Nursing*, 11(5): 583–8.

Roberts M (2007) Modernity, mental illness and the crisis of meaning. *Journal of Psychiatric and Mental Health Nursing*, 14(3): 277–81.

Roberts M (2008) Facilitating recovery by making sense of suffering: a Nietzschean perspective. *Journal of Psychiatric and Mental Health Nursing*, 15(9): 743–8.

Roberts M (2010) Service user involvement and the restrictive sense of psychiatric categories: the challenge facing mental health nurses. *Journal of Psychiatric and Mental Health Nursing*, 17(4): 289–94.

Roberts M (2014) Beyond the bounds of the dogmatic image of thought: the development of critical, creative thinking in the mental health professions. *Journal of Psychiatric and Mental Health Nursing*, 21(4): 313–19.

Roberts M & Ion R (2015) Thinking critically about the occurrence of widespread participation in poor nursing care. *Journal of Advanced Nursing*, 71(4): 768–76.

Roberts M & Lamont E (2014) Suicide: an existentialist reconceptualization. *Journal of Psychiatric and Mental Health Nursing*, 21(10): 873–8.

Robertson D (2010) *The Philosophy of Cognitive-Behavioural Therapy: Stoic philosophy as rational and cognitive psychotherapy*. London: Karnac Books.

Rogers A & Pilgrim D (2014) *A Sociology of Mental Health and Illness*, 5th edition. Maidenhead: Open University Press.

Rogers CR (1957) The necessary and sufficient conditions of therapeutic personality change. *Journal of Consulting Psychology*, 21(2): 95–103.

Rogers CR (2004/1961) *On Becoming a Person: A therapist's view of psychotherapy*. London: Constable.

Rolfe G (2011) Models and frameworks for critical reflection, in Rolfe G, Jasper M & Freshwater D (eds) *Critical Reflection in Practice*, 2nd edition. Basingstoke: Palgrave Macmillan, pp. 31–51.

Rolfe G, Jasper M & Freshwater D (eds) (2011) *Critical Reflection in Practice: Generating knowledge for care*, 2nd edition. Basingstoke: Palgrave Macmillan.

Romme M & Escher S (eds) (1993) *Accepting Voices*. London: Mind Publications.

Romme M & Escher S (2000) *Making Sense of Voices: A guide for mental health professionals working with voice-hearers*. London: Mind Publications.

Rose D, Thornicroft G, Pinfold V & Kassam A (2007) 250 labels used to stigmatise people with mental illness. *BMC Health Services Research*, 7: 97.

Ross CA & Goldner EM (2009) Stigma, negative attitudes and discrimination towards mental illness within the nursing profession: a review of the literature. *Journal of Psychiatric and Mental Health Nursing*, 16(6): 558–67.

Sackett DL, Rosenberg WMC, Muir Gray JA, Haynes RB & Richardson WS (1996) Evidence-based medicine: what it is and what it isn't. *British Medical Journal*, 312: 71–2.

Said EW (1978) *Orientalism.* London: Routledge & Kegan Paul.

Santa Mina E & Gallop R (2009) The person who is suicidal, in Barker P (ed) *Psychiatric and Mental Health Nursing: The craft of caring*, 2nd edition. London: Hodder Arnold, pp. 182–90.

Scheff TJ (2009/1966) *Being Mentally Ill: A sociological theory*, 3rd edition. Piscataway, NJ: Transaction Publishers.

Schön DA (1983) *The Reflective Practitioner: How professionals think in action.* New York: Basic Books.

Scottish Executive (2006) *Rights, Relationships and Recovery: The report of the national review of mental health nursing in Scotland.* Edinburgh: Scottish Executive.

Scull A (2011) *Madness: A very short introduction.* Oxford: Oxford University Press.

Scull A (2015) *Madness in Civilization: A cultural history of insanity from the Bible to Freud, from the madhouse to modern medicine.* London: Thames & Hudson.

Sellars J (2006) *Stoicism.* Chesham: Acumen.

Shepherd G, Boardman J & Slade M (2008) *Making Recovery a Reality.* London: Sainsbury Centre for Mental Health.

Shorter E (1997) *A History of Psychiatry: From the era of the asylum to the age of Prozac.* New York: John Wiley.

Showalter E (1987) *The Female Malady: Women, madness and English culture, 1830–1980.* London: Virago.

Smail D (2005) *Power, Interest and Psychology: Elements of a social materialist understanding of distress.* Ross-on-Wye: PCCS Books.

Stacey G & Diamond B (2014) Values in practice, in Stickley T & Wright N (eds) *Theories for Mental Health Nursing: A guide for practice.* London: Sage, pp. 235–50.

Stickley T (2006) Should service user involvement be consigned to history? A critical realist perspective. *Journal of Psychiatric and Mental Health Nursing*, 13(5): 570–7.

Stickley T & Spandler H (2014) Compassion and mental health nursing, in Stickley T & Wright N (eds) *Theories for Mental Health Nursing: A guide for practice.* London: Sage, pp. 134–46.

Stringer B, Van Meijel B, De Vree W & Van Der Bijl J (2008) User involvement in mental health care: the role of nurses. A literature review. *Journal of Psychiatric and Mental Health Nursing*, 15(8): 678–83.

Strother E, Lemberg R, Stanford SC & Turberville D (2012) Eating disorders in men: underdiagnosed, undertreated, and misunderstood. *Eating Disorders*, 20(5): 346–55.

Swatridge C (2014) *Oxford Guide to Effective Argument and Critical Thinking.* Oxford: Oxford University Press.

Szasz TS (1961) *The Myth of Mental Illness: Foundations of a theory of personal conduct.* New York: Paul B. Hoeber.

Szasz TS (1983) The myth of mental illness, in Szasz T (ed) *Ideology and Insanity: Essays on the psychiatric dehumanization of man.* London: Marion Boyars, pp. 12–24.

Taylor BJ (2010) *Reflective Practice for Healthcare Professionals: A practical guide*, 3rd edition. Maidenhead: Open University Press.

Taylor DB (2013) *Writing Skills for Nursing and Midwifery Students.* London: Sage.

Tee S & Lathlean JA (2012) Appraising and using evidence in mental health practice, in Tee S, Brown J & Carpenter D (eds) *Handbook of Mental Health Nursing.* London: Hodder Arnold, pp. 121–38.

Thompson S & Thompson N (2008) *The Critically Reflective Practitioner.* Basingstoke: Palgrave Macmillan.

Thornicroft G (2006) *Shunned: Discrimination against people with mental illness.* Oxford: Oxford University Press.

Turton W (2015) An introduction to psychosocial interventions, in Walker S (ed) *Psychosocial Interventions in Mental Health Nursing.* London: Sage/Learning Matters, pp. 4–21.

Ussher JM (1991) *Women's Madness: Misogyny or mental illness?* Hemel Hempstead: Harvester Wheatsheaf.

Walker S (ed) (2014) *Engagement and Therapeutic Communication in Mental Health Nursing.* London: Sage/ Learning Matters.

Walker S (ed) (2015) *Psychosocial Interventions in Mental Health Nursing.* London: Sage/Learning Matters.

Wallace M & Wray A (2013) *Critical Reading and Writing for Postgraduates,* 2nd edition. London: Sage.

Walsh M (2009) (Mis)representing mental distress? in Reynolds J, Muston R, Heller T, Leach J, McCormick M, Wallcraft J & Walsh M (eds) *Mental Health Still Matters.* Basingstoke: Palgrave Macmillan, pp. 135–40.

Wampold BE & Imel ZE (2015) *The Great Psychotherapy Debate: The evidence for what makes psychotherapy work,* 2nd edition. Hove: Routledge.

Warner S & Wilkins T (2003) Diagnosing distress and reproducing disorder: women, child sexual abuse and 'borderline personality disorder', in Reavey P & Warner S (eds) *New Feminist Stories of Childhood Sexual Abuse: Sexual scripts and dangerous dialogues.* London: Routledge, pp. 167–86.

Watters E (2011) *Crazy Like Us: The globalization of the Western mind.* London: Constable & Robinson.

Weinstein J (ed) (2010) *Mental Health, Service User Involvement and Recovery.* London: Jessica Kingsley.

Weston A (2009) *A Rulebook for Arguments,* 4th edition. Indianapolis: Hackett.

Westwood L & Baker J (2010) Attitudes and perceptions of mental health nurses towards borderline personality disorder clients in acute mental health settings: a review of the literature. *Journal of Psychiatric and Mental Health Nursing,* 17(7): 657–62.

White S, Fook J & Gardner F (eds) (2006) *Critical Reflection in Health and Social Care.* Maidenhead: Open University Press.

WHO (World Health Organization) (1992) *The ICD-10 Classification of Mental and Behavioural Disorders: Clinical descriptions and diagnostic guidelines.* Geneva: WHO.

WHO (World Health Organization) (2014) *Social Determinants of Mental Health.* Geneva: WHO.

Williams M, Teasdale J, Segal Z & Kabat-Zinn J (2007) *The Mindful Way Through Depression: Freeing yourself from chronic unhappiness.* New York: The Guilford Press.

Winship G & Hardy S (2014) Counselling and psychotherapy in mental health nursing: therapeutic encounters, in Stickley T & Wright N (eds) *Theories for Mental Health Nursing: A guide for practice.* London: Sage, pp. 223–34.

Woolliams M, Williams K, Butcher D & Pye J (2011) *Be More Critical! A practical guide for health and social care students,* 2nd edition. Oxford: Oxford Brookes University.

Wright K, Haigh K & McKeown M (2007) Reclaiming the humanity in personality disorder. *International Journal of Mental Health Nursing,* 16(4): 236–46.

Young Minds (2010) *Stigma: A review of the evidence.* London: Young Minds.

Zubin J & Spring B (1977) Vulnerability: a new view of schizophrenia. *Journal of Abnormal Psychology,* 86(2): 103–26.

Index